SPRINGER SERIES ON INDUSTRY AND HEALTH CARE
NUMBER 2

W0227759

A Business Perspective on Industry and Health Care

Willis B. Goldbeck

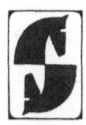

Springer-Verlag   New York Heidelberg Berlin

Richard H. Egdahl, M.D., Ph.D.
Center for Industry and Health Care
Boston University Health Policy Institute
53 Bay State Road
Boston, Massachusetts 02215

Library of Congress Cataloging in Publication Data

Goldbeck, Willis.
    A business perspective on industry and health care.

    (Springer series on industry and health care; no. 2) 1. Labor and laboring classes—Medical care—United States. 2. Medical policy—United States. I. Title.
HD7102.U5G64   362.1'0973   77-17982

9 8 7 6 5 4 3 2 1

ISBN-13: 978-0-387-90298-2   e-ISBN-13: 978-1-4612-6270-1
DOI: 10.1007/978-1-4612-6270-1

Foreword

The Springer Series on Industry and Health Care is intended to characterize present and future ways in which industry can influence the nation's health care system in the direction of greater efficiency and effectiveness. Its potential audience includes nearly everyone interested in health care because the system's future configuration is now being influenced by corporate health programs and the involvement of individual corporate leaders in health affairs.

The first volume of the Springer Series provided a broad background on industry as a payer, provider, and consumer of health services. Unlike volumes planned for the future, it did not single out any particular aspect of corporate activity in health but rather identified and catalogued the many new involvements of industry, both management and labor, in the health care scene.

This, the second volume in the series, is designed to complement the first and to complete the process of laying the groundwork for the series as a whole. Volume two covers the same vista as volume one, but paints with a broader brush. It seemed to us, as editors of the series and authors of volume one, that the academic and somewhat distant overview we provided could be rounded out in a second volume by someone with a more immediate and practical perspective on industry's involvement in health care.

Accordingly, we asked Willis B. Goldbeck, executive director of the Washington Business Group on Health, to put together his thoughts on industry and health policy, drawing both on his personal experience and on his participation in our first conference on industry and health care, held in Boston on June 4–5, 1977. With the aid of a grant from the Robert Wood Johnson

Foundation, that conference brought together representatives from a variety of industries for a vigorous exchange of ideas. Mr. Goldbeck has worked some portions of it into his presentation, but has made no attempt at encyclopedic coverage. Conference participants all received advance copies of eighteen specially prepared background papers. These comprise the third volume of the Springer Series, which touches upon corporate health programs, prepaid health plans, corporate liability, union health clinics, occupational health and safety, and a wide range of related issues.

In this volume, Mr. Goldbeck writes from the experience of several years in Washington, the last three working closely with corporate leadership to focus industry attention on legislation and policy issues related to health. The perspective is his own and represents an important outlook at this juncture while the Springer Series is establishing baselines of knowledge on current industrial health programs and potential developments for the future.

We anticipate that future volumes of the series will adhere more closely to the conferences on which they draw, and will present the variety of different points of view expressed by conference participants on critical topics. Their focus will thus be narrower than that of the first two volumes. The fourth volume will build on our November 1977 conference "Employee and Employer Decisions about Health: Informational Issues." Future conferences and volumes in the series will seek to provide in-depth analysis of further health-related topics of importance to industry.

Boston, September 1977

Richard H. Egdahl
Series Editor

Diana Chapman Walsh
Assistant Editor

Preface

This monograph is not a research document but one individual's perspective on the major issues related to industry and health care. My thoughts have grown out of the past three years of work in Washington, extensive travel throughout the country, work here and abroad on other public policy issues, and most recently, my participation with the Boston University Health Policy Institute's growing Center for Industry and Health Care.

Business interest in health care ranges widely, as do my thoughts in this monograph. I have tried to extract from my interactions with business and government leaders, as well as from the center's June 1977 conference, some general principles and observations that I feel might be of some interest and use to those in industry who are becoming involved in the complex health policy arena and to those who are contemplating such involvement.

Industry's role in health policy formulation is rather new and thus neither cohesive nor comprehensive. Yet great progress has been made in the past few years and there does appear to be a recognition, grudging from some, of industry as a force—now and in the future—that must be reckoned with in health policy. That, however, is just step one. The real test will be in the way industry responds to these new opportunities.

There exist many examples of employers acting as the key change agents at the local level to bring about more cost-effective medical care delivery without any reduction in the quality of that care. At the federal level, industry is slowly becoming a respected participant, but it is not yet clear either how much of a long-term effort industry is willing to make or how seriously the government is taking the effort now expended. But I am convinced that the United States cannot have a successful national health insurance program of any kind without the informed support and involvement of industry.

This monograph is dedicated to those in industry who were toiling in the trenches before it was fashionable to do so, before even their own companies, in many cases, recognized the importance of their efforts. They constitute a resource that industry, government, and providers cannot afford to ignore in the formulation of future health policy.

As with all such ventures, this monograph benefited greatly from the efforts of many. I am especially grateful to the team at the Boston University Health Policy Institute, to the staff of the Washington Business Group on Health, to Jan Jennings who is my personal source of strength, and, most importantly, to those in industry who have given me the opportunity to share in their work.

Washington, D.C., September 1977   Willis B. Goldbeck

Contents

Introduction

1

When one category of our nation's expenditures increases at a pace far more rapid than most others, when the total spent for that category approaches $160 billion a year or nearly 9 percent of our gross national product, and when that category happens to directly affect the life of every single person in the United States, it is only reasonable for all factions in the public and private sectors to examine the situation. Such examinations usually become a search for someone to blame.

This is the case with the current concern for our health care system. The huge amount of money being spent on what we generally call health and the rate at which that amount has been escalating (double every five years or less) have led to two predictable reactions: first, the assumption that something must be wrong, and therefore we (government and the private sector) must find solutions; and second, that to deal with a problem of this magnitude, we must single out the largest elements of the financing and delivery systems, rather than attempting to address the problem as a whole. Not everyone agrees that this segmented, or phased, approach is best but it is the approach that is prevailing.

There is general agreement that, indeed, something is wrong. There is much less agreement on the magnitude of the problem and its possible solutions. This arises from the basic fact that there is no health budget and therefore no orderly mechanism for assessing the amount that we *should* be spending. There is no known correct percentage of GNP that should be applied to health and there is no process for determining one. Economists generally seem to agree that 9 percent is too high in relation to all the other things we demand with our limited fiscal resources, but none can say what the right amount should be.

The United States has the capacity to provide much of the medical care our population wants, but only at the expense of some of those other things that we say we also want. Since the demand for medical services appears to be insatiable, pressures increasingly bear on the political system to provide a priority-setting mechanism—a way to determine how much of our resources we allocate to health care and how much to other things. This is further complicated by the fact that health, and even medical care, is not a discrete program or issue that can be described and financed in isolation. Substantial portions of our health care expenditures purchase transportation, help counteract local unemployment, improve or make available shelter, and otherwise overlap with other program and service categories.

In its simplest terms, much of our current health policy debate concerns the rationing of health and medical care. Distasteful as it may be, rationing is inevitable. Resources are limited. Competition among all worthwhile expenditures is increasing and our population is both increasing and getting older, guaranteeing further increases in demand. The implication should be clear. Unless we are willing to accept a declining capacity for quality health and medical care, we must make better use of the resources available.

Industry's emerging role in health policy is predicated on the realization that industry must have an influence on the decisions that will be made for future allocations of health resources. This is true regardless of the fate of national health insurance in the United States. As a consumer/provider/purchaser of health insurance and medical care, industry has an economic stake estimated to exceed $35 billion in 1977, and that does not even include lost time, death benefits, retraining, health education programs, workmen's compensation, etc.

Today, industry is trying to recover from three decades during which it signed premium checks, contributed with great civic pride to hospitals regardless of need, and rarely questioned the right of the provider to dictate the terms as well as the content and methods of care to be delivered. Further, the growing government intervention in the health system during that time aroused almost no interest, concern, or involvement, pro or con, on the part of industry.

The price for this acquiescence is enormous. Companies find their health insurance premiums going up 100 percent while their health benefits expand, on average, less than 20 percent. Waste and duplication characterize a medical delivery system that has been allowed to fill in a virtual blank check against industry's account. Health education and promotion have received minimal attention. And, most disappointing of all, there is little to indicate that the vast cost increases have led to a concomitant increase in the health status of our population. Industry's new role in health policy is one of throwing off the habit of acquiescence and becoming an informed, assertive participant. Industry has a clear objective: to reform our private health care system so that it might survive.

Fully cognizant of the important role government plays today (it, too, is a consumer, provider, and payer of grand proportions, as well as the regulater), industry is committed to a balance between the best qualities of the private and public systems for the long-term benefit of all. Central to this philosophy is the theme that the health care system is entirely too large, complex, and costly to have its design, finance, and management successfully handled by one sector of society to the exclusion of the other.

In this monograph, the term *industry* is used to mean private sector employers of all kinds. The focus, however, is on those very large firms whose employment and purchasing power are so extensive that their private decisions concerning health care benefits become public decisions affecting the economics of the entire health delivery system.

Where appropriate, labor is included within this general definition of *industry*. For example, those unions that provide their members' health benefits through their own insurance programs and those that actually deliver medical care have the same economic incentives, concerns, and potential influence as management. Also, the health-related decisions of management, especially in the very large firms, derive to a substantial degree from the collective bargaining process. This is particularly important because it explains, in part, why industry has been slow to become involved in the health care cost debate. Typically in the big companies, those costs, however large, are but a small portion of the total compensation package.

Labor has, since World War II, pressed management and government to steadily expand the coverage and size of health benefits, while pressing simultaneously to reduce the cost to the worker of these benefits. Therefore, labor must share with management the blame for contributing to the economic incentives that cause providers to drive health care costs upward at a pace beyond what can be explained by either normal inflation or increased utilization based on need.

The increasing involvement of industry (including labor) in the health policy arena has been in part stimulated by, and is also serving as a catalyst for, direct action at the local level. Whether it is manifested by participation on the board of a health systems agency, the establishment of a preadmission testing program, or innovative health education program, or the expansion of the corporate medical facility to a full care system for the workers and their families, industry's increased capacity to become a respected voice in health policy has combined with the pressure of increasing health care costs to alter, in many cases dramatically, industry's position as payer, provider, and consumer of medical care.

No sector of our society—not government, academia, the health professions, or industry—is united on the best way to solve our health care problems. This monograph will explore the various corporate action programs as well as the expanding role of industry in health policy.

Health Is More Than Medical Care

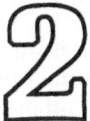

The general public seems convinced that contemporary medicine is able to accomplish a great deal more than is in fact possible.[1]

Industry is bringing itself to the health policy table just at the time when the issues on the table are at a peak of complexity and controversy. The cost issue has forced an investigation of the health industry by more examiners and in greater detail than ever before. Three themes seem to dominate the results of these examinations. First, health care programs and insurance are concerned primarily with curative medicine, not health. Not only is this bad from the standpoint of the health status of our population, it is also a major contributor to cost problems. We spend amazing sums curing what could have been prevented for a pittance, or even through simple awareness and motivation. Second, health, far more than medical care, is inextricably linked with many other social policy sectors. Transportation, housing, the environment, employment, and individual life-style are the primary health determinants. John

Knowles expresses it: "Health care is only one element in the quality of life equation." Others do as well:

> To make matters worse, there is the perverse human knack for creating new problems in the very process of solving old ones. Mastering our own environment, we endanger ourselves by polluting it. Becoming affluent, we subject ourselves to the stresses of a crowded, fast-moving world, and at the same time allow ourselves to slip into a dangerously sedentary way of life, eating, drinking, and smoking to excess. Achieving mobility, we kill and maim each other with our motor cars. Relieved of much physical ill-health, whole vistas of mental distress open before us. And when by standards of the less fortunate, we are relatively free from definable mental or physical ill-health, we become less able than our ancestors to endure minor complaints.[2]

The third theme is simple to state but even more difficult than the previous two to resolve. Basic to the design of national health insurance or even a non-NHI long-range cost containment strategy is the need to reach agreement on how much money we as a nation feel should be allocated to the broad category of health. Only then will it be possible to design an allocation process than can, and we hope will, lead to better health outcomes with fewer wasted resources. These three issues pose a series of complex problems and opportunities for industry.

The contradictions between industry's reason for being, that is, to make a profit, and industry's responsibilities in the health area are numerous. The work setting is a most dangerous place, yet only industry can implement the Occupational Safety and Health Act; the health care industry itself is a giant employer in an era of serious unemployment, yet we are asking it to become more efficient and less labor intensive; cigarette manufacturers are concerned with the ravages of alcoholism, while the liquor industry notes the impact of smoking on health yet both are understandably reluctant to acknowledge the health effects of their own products; a new plant cannot be built because of air pollution regulations, yet the old plant cannot be modernized to meet noise pollution regulations. The list is endless and frustrating, yet for now perhaps inevitable. We are a society struggling to set priorities and meet self-imposed new standards of suitability for our working and living environments.

Industry cannot resolve these problems alone, but it clearly must be part of the process of resolution. As a society considering national health insurance, we must recognize that costs cannot be sufficiently contained nor health status sufficiently improved unless these issues are addressed and the programmatic overlaps recognized between health, shelter, transportation, employment, and the environment. This is not a new message, but it is now being brought to the attention of key decision-makers with increasing regularity.

For example, a National Health Insurance Advisory Committee to HEW's Secretary, Joseph Califano, has, in 1977, visited a variety of communities across the country to view and hear presentations on specific health delivery problems and programs. By traveling with that committee as an observer, I have been able to gain a series of impressions that form a mosaic of the nonmedical aspects of our health delivery problems. It is hard to avoid the conclusion that these problems are more concerned with delivery than with health. Some examples may be useful.

Watts, Los Angeles. While all the area's problems derive from overall economic depression, several specific issues exemplify the difficulty of trying to resolve health delivery problems through a focus on medical care. Rick Carlson has suggested that the health industry be looked upon primarily as an employer: that could be appropriate for Watts. When HEW reduced funding for the Watts Health Foundation, some one hundred employees were laid off. Local observers recall the impact of this upon the community at large as the closest they have come to a repetition of the riots of the late 1960s. Yet despite a staff reduction of this magnitude, no one with whom I spoke indicated that there had been any consequent reduction in the quality of medical care delivered. The problem clearly arose from the extramedical role of the foundation as the second largest employer in Watts.

Another nonmedical problem is transportation. Owing to the absence of public transportation, a major item in the foundation's budget is their own service of transporting patients to and from the clinics and the hospital. A third problem is the political and professional squabbling between the foundation and the Martin Luther King Hospital. As a result, the foundation refers patients to the Los Angeles County Hospital, which is already overcrowded and much farther away, thus exacerbating the transportation problem.

East Los Angeles. Many who visited the Hispanic clinic came away with the feeling that its primary reason for being was language translation. The clinic is able to provide an atmosphere in which the local Spanish-speaking residents feel they are treated with dignity and can be understood, not just in terms of spoken or written word but also in terms of their cultural needs and traditions.

Los Angeles County Hospital. The problems here, and they appear to be typical of large government hospitals elsewhere, are, from the patient's point of view, the style of delivery. The impersonal treatment that results from the massive scale of the institution, the fact that it is the last resort for many of the patients, and the fact that the question of the quality of care is overwhelmed by the complexities and inconsistencies of management all give rise to complaints. There is little doubt that the physicians do care, but there is little time for them to practice the gentle art of caring.

From the hospital's point of view, the problems are ones of management: lost records, union problems, and the problems caused by the lack of continuity of government program funding and direction. The latter were stressed at every location visited by the Advisory Committee and are just as important for the development of new technology in Yale's clinical laboratory as for the delivery of primary care in rural America.

San Antonio. Again, transportation and lack of program continuity are the major problems. For the migrant workers in the surrounding area, management is not a problem because there is no medical care system to be managed. Epitomizing the issue of maldistribution of physicians the migrant areas have no resident physicians. The clinic, impressive for all that is being attempted and the high degree of caring that was evident, nonetheless is totally dependent on funds from Washington and survives on dedication rather than medical or professional resources.

All these problems do have an impact on the quality of care delivered, or at least on the patient's perception of quality, but none is itself amenable to a medical solution. All must be addressed from a broader perspective and looked upon as factors that need improvement in order to allow the quality of care to be maintained, let alone improved.

It is not necessary to limit this examination to specific communities. When the focus is shifted to particular health issues, nonmedical factors remain important. Mental health care does not suffer from lack of medical or technical capacity: mental problems are not treated at a level commensurate with their importance because treatment is, in most cases, not covered by insurance. They are not treated because there remains a stigma attached to anyone who is identified as having mental problems. The delivery problems in this area are the result of the reimbursement system and of societal values which are slow to change.

Nutrition is another example. We know that our eating habits are a basic determinant of our health. We know that a very large amount of the illness that our medical system is asked to treat results from foods that are bad and habits that are worse. There is little our medical system can do about this.

The same can be said for health education. It is not taught in the schools and only obliquely referred to even in medical education. For most of our lives we receive every possible stimulus to act in ways that are contrary to the maintenance of good health. We pay the price in teenage pregnancy, VD, obesity, hypertension, alcoholism, and so on. In addition, few among us are taught how best to use the medical resources our insurance and financial wherewithal make available.

It is precisely these facts, as well as the ever-broadening context of the health system, that make health costs so hard to contain. We have arrived at an annual expenditure of approximately $160 billion dollars for what we call health care. But we did not do so by deciding that $160 billion was what we needed to spend, or because we knew what we were getting, or even because we liked the results of what we bought. It just happened, incrementally, with many influencing factors and no one source to either blame or praise. The issue facing the administration, Congress, the professions, the public, and, more than ever before, industry, is how much do we want to spend and for what? Nearly everyone agrees that if we took the $160 billion and somehow reallocated it to meet the optimal health objectives, we would not replicate the system we now have. But there is little agreement on what a new system would look like or what elements of the existing system would be eliminated.

In all these themes and their many problem areas, industry is a critical element. The challenge for the next decade will be to see if there can be forged a public-private partnership for better health. Industry must consciously use its vast reimbursement power as an agent for change and must take an increasing role in the direct delivery of care. Industry must also provide educational programs and incentives for employees and their families to alter their personal behavior. And, industry must take a leadership role in the design and adaptation of the new environmental, living, and working standards our society indicates it desires.

We will not, I predict, have a single health budget in the United States in the foreseeable future. And we will certainly not have all our conflicting policies and programs rationalized. But even with these difficulties, we can make the philosophical change and programmatic commitment to move from the medical model to a health model. Within that process of reorientation, conventional medicine can and should be expected to play a major role and to continue to pursue excellence. But it will do so within a broader context that recognizes, as the highest priority, health and its maintenance.

Health Policy: A New Arena for Industry

3

Historically, industry chose to leave health policy largely in the hands of the providers. As government began to finance and regulate more and more of the health care industry, business still undertook little involvement. Uncomfortable about appearing to tell another sector of the free enterprise system what to do, industry also held the medical profession in almost mythical deference. Hospitals were charity—symbols of community pride whose presence and growth were laudable without regard to need. Physicians were the symbol of the American entrepreneur often battling alone against the endless intrusions of big government. Industry paid its insurance premiums and built its in-plant clinics, but it entered the policy arena only when government began to regulate health and safety in industry itself.

Somewhere in the early 1970s a few business leaders began to notice a number of problems which, today, we know are interrelated. The productivity of the average worker was declining. The utilization and the cost of medical benefits was going up—fast. Government was rapidly becoming the dominant force in medical care financing, a fact that carried with it the implication of ever-growing regulation. At the same time, old health problems, now defeated, were replaced by new, or newly identified, and more complex and costly problems that were not amenable to traditional therapy—environmental contamination, drug dependency, stress, obesity, and so on. Two time-honored motivators, uncertainty (of government regulation and national health insurance) and money (the increasing cost of employer-purchased medical care and the potential cost of NHI) led industry to reexamine its traditional role—and seek a new role.

Industry's expanded involvement must, however, be viewed in the proper context. Foremost is the simple fact that there is no such thing as *the* business community. Congress has known this for years; business, generally, is just becoming willing to accept it and live with its own inherent conflicts. This monograph focuses on the major employers, to whom I refer as "business" or "industry." It is usually the small number of giants who influence policy for the larger number of smaller organizations in any policy area; health will be no exception. But that does not mean that the policy outcome best for the biggest employers is necessarily best for industry as a whole, or for the rest of us.

Second, some employers have been responsibly involved in HMOs, expanded clinics, planning, and so forth for many years. This is easily overlooked when speaking of industry involvement as a phenomenon of the 1970s. Yet even today, many companies have not felt the economic pinch strongly enough to warrant giving health and medical care a high priority. Third, there is no simple solution or single path industry should take in health and medical care. The problems, their costs, and the opportunities are all so vast that they can accommodate a broad range of well-intentioned remedial efforts.

Fourth, business leaders are generally isolated from personal exposure to our nation's medical care problem. Their involvement, then, is in proportion to their understanding of overall societal problems and of how those adversely affect their companies. Finally, industry has no desire to leave its comfortable, supportive relationship with the provider professions. To the extent that industry does shift to an adversary posture or to providing more direct care, it will be indicting organized medicine for failure to keep pace with the changing needs of those it serves.

The chronology of industry involvement in health policy tends to parallel the new, more enlightened industry attitudes toward public policy in general. Business had earned itself the unenviable reputation of being predominently negative, of opposing all governmental action. Starting in the early 1970s and especially in the aftermath of the Nixon White House disgrace, much of industry has attempted to work more closely with government and to attempt positive contributions to public policy decision-making. Leading this new approach is The Business Roundtable, an organization comprising the chief executives of approximately 178 major corporations, and their Health Task Force, chaired by Charles J. Pilliod, Jr., Chairman of the Board, Goodyear Tire & Rubber Company.

In August 1974 the Washington Business Group on Health (WBGH) was born in this spirit of constructive cooperation. From a nucleus of 5 companies, the WBGH has grown to a current membership of 150. Significantly, these relatively few companies provide the health care benefits for more than 30 million employees, retirees, and dependents. Separately, these companies have a varied, but local, impact on health policy. In the aggregate, with their multiple roles as payers, providers, and consumers of health care services, they represent an awesome resource that policymakers can ill-afford to ignore.

To have the policymakers in Washington, and increasingly at the state level, use industry as a resource, several progressive steps had to be achieved. First, companies had to be convinced that in fact they were a valuable resource. Second, a process of information-gathering had to be established. It had to be anticipatory as well as reactive, and it had to be fast to provide timely data for the rapidly changing political and legislative process.

Perhaps most important, credibility had to be developed and maintained. To serve as a legitimate resource, industry-generated information had to be accurate, nonpartisan, and supported by industry experts whose commitment included personal participation. Further, although unabashedly desirous of influencing the future direction of health policy, industry needed a vehicle for involvement that differentiated itself from traditional corporate lobbying organizations and tactics. The theory was, and is, that if the industry resource is valid, its presence will be felt through substantive work. Finally, that substantive work could not be limited to the "headline" issues like national health insurance. Indeed, to gain the level of respect necessary to have an impact on these issues, the industry resource had to be applied to many immediate and, by comparison, smaller health care issues.

The WBGH was established to implement the program just described. During its three years, it has become a recognized factor in extending and deepening the acceptance of industry as a resource in health policy. This is not the place (and I am certainly not the person) to evaluate the WBGH's progress or isolate its accomplishments from other positive influences that have been felt in the past three years. What can be done, however, is to note some of the important but little known ways that industry is involved today.

Before the involvement of industry the National High Blood Pressure Education Program (NHBPEP) of the National Institutes of Health had great success in alerting the public to the dangers of hypertension and in reducing the number of unknowing victims but was less successful in starting and maintaining people on treatment programs once they had been diagnosed. The disease is frequently asymptomatic and the medication can actually make patients feel worse than they did before. In this case "feeling worse" may actually mean "getting better," but that is a hard story to sell to even the most receptive patient. Add the fact that the patients must take the medication every day for the rest of their lives and it is easy to see why maintenance rates are not high. In 1977 the NHBPEP initiated a special program in the work setting, because this setting can be viewed as a major communications channel for reaching millions who might otherwise go unscreened and untreated. Industry is included on its steering committee and employers are working with the government, labor, and provider groups to develop new methods of improving treatment maintenance rates.

A Center for Industry and Health Care has been established within the

Boston University Health Policy Institute by Richard H. Egdahl, M.D., in conjunction with the WBGH and individual corporations. This center's program, of which the Springer Series and the related conferences are elements, will provide technical and analytical resources and will work with industry as the new industrial roles in health care policy and delivery mature.

Employers, working with voluntary health organizations led by the American Public Health Association and with foreign ministries of health, have established the International Health Resource Consortium (IHRC) to serve as a coordinating mechanism for efforts to improve health services delivery in developing countries. Its distinguishing feature, in addition to the unusual cooperation of its founding organizations, will be its emphasis on assisting the indigenous population to identify their own needs and then form a local counterpart consortium to work for solutions. IHRC will not be a giveaway program. It will, if successful, be a catalyst for improved health care and more effective allocation of corporate health benefits and program resources.

The National Institute of Mental Health, in recognition of the growing role taken by employers, has established a new study group, with industry participation, to address the special problems and opportunities afforded by employment-based mental health programs and benefits. At the same time, employers in cooperation with the Health Insurance Association of America, have been working at the state level in Maryland and California to improve and expand hospital rate review and concurrent utilization review programs. During the coming year, this effort will be expanded to other states, enlarging the network of participating employers. These are informal projects involving labor, all types of insurance carriers, the local hospitals and medical associations, and local public officials.

The economic incentives inherent in so many employee benefit plans are being changed to use the reimbursement system to encourage more cost-effective treatment procedures. These include outpatient care, ambulatory surgi-centers, second surgical opinion experiments, covered mental health treatment, concurrent utilization review for all classes of patients, use of paramedics and other forms of physician extenders, home health care, preventive examinations, procedures, and behavioral change clinics (alcoholism, smoking, off-work safety, and so on), better utilization (which can often mean less utilization) of existing benefits, and utilization of major equipment and facilities only if they have been approved by the local planning system. None of these progressive steps is free or even cheap. One measure of industry's involvement is their recognition that the types of major change being sought in our health care system cannot be achieved overnight or without a substantial commitment by the major purchasers.

Another indication of industry's growing involvement is the willingness of congressional and administration health policymakers to call upon the WBGH to assemble groups of industry executives for open dialogue on a wide variety of topics. The most recent issue discussed was the development of an international health policy that would have an impact on multinational corporations. A second issue was the relationship between employee benefit programs and the health care cost impact of medical technology. Of particular interest was the potential use of insurance reimbursement restrictions as a mechanism to control the proliferation of technology that has not been approved through the planning system's certificate of need process or for which there has not yet been sufficient assessment to assure the user of its effectiveness.

Industry's involvement with health policy is occurring on several levels simultaneously. Between efforts to influence policy on the federal level and to alter corporate policies of benefit design, industry-sponsored health services are having an impact upon the cost and delivery of care at the state and local levels. These are the subject of the next chapter.

Health Planning and Resource Allocation

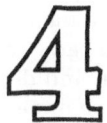

Health planning is not going to save big money today, or even tomorrow, but it is a rational start to get some sense of efficiency into the system. We support HSAs because we believe there is a tremendous amount of waste in the health care system.

Richard Martin

Health planning is not new. P.L. 93–641, the National Health Planning and Resources Development Act, established the current planning system with local health systems agencies (HSAs) as its base. It was an outgrowth of decades of private and public attempts to impose some order on our medical care system. I say *medical care* because, despite its title, the law really has little to do with health. It is a regulatory process for the planning of medical care facilities. In simpler terms, it is a process for rationing limited resources in the face of insatiable demand.

As the new planning system has evolved, it has taken on several characteristics that distinguish it from its ineffective predecessors, aside from its greater comprehensiveness. First, certificate of need programs make the planner also the regulator. Future developments of this approach will be much stronger, requiring recertification of existing facilities and decertification of those no longer serving their intended purpose. Second, consumers, rather than providers, have majority control of the HSAs. This is not working in every instance, in part because providers resist any loss of authority and in part because there are too few well-informed consumers with time to devote to the process. HSA directors frequently report that the providers have a real majority at most meetings.

But two precedents are vital. First, the definition of *consumer* clearly includes the major purchasers of medical care. Therefore, industry and labor sit together on the consumer advocacy side of the table. Second, provider expertise is essential in an advisory but not necessarily a policy making role. The "super" cardiologist or hospital administrator is no longer looked to automatically as the final voice on setting priorities for community health care.

Industry's Role

The HSAs are an excellent vehicle for industry not only to become involved but also to make a major contribution to reshaping local medical care delivery. Industry has always been a principal payer for medical care. Corporations paid their health insurance premiums with little question and designed their benefit plans with economic incentives inevitably producing unnecessary hospitalization. Corporate officers served on hospital boards but did so more as philanthropists than as businesspeople. Contributions were given to finance new and expanded facilities to meet the demand that their employee health benefits had in part stimulated. The demands of physicians for new equipment and facilities were rarely questioned by the industry representatives of the board.

> If you are going to get involved, you have to develop a different point of view in dealing with hospitals. They are not the United Way or Community Chest. They are institutions that are providing a service and are costing your company a lot of money.
>
> Richard Martin

Today, there is a new spirit and purpose to corporate involvement. Health insurance plans are being redesigned to change the emphasis to noninstitutional forms of care. Businesspeople are increasingly acting like businesspeople while serving on hospital boards, and corporate leaders are less reluctant to express, publicly, great concern over the conduct of providers and medical institutions. This can be illustrated by an excerpt from remarks by Goodyear's chairman, Charles J. Pilliod, Jr., delivered to the annual meeting of the American Hospital Association on August 31, 1977.

I think you must face the reality that overall, hospitals and health care are not as efficient as they could be, and you administrators should be asking yourselves some searching questions about your performance.

When you compete with one another in the community to have the latest equipment, rather than looking at the community equipment needs as a whole, you are not doing a good job as administrators.

If your institution does not have a legitimate 90 percent occupancy rate, with proper concurrent utilization controls, you are not doing a good job.

If you let the pressures from your medical staff distort your presentation of facts to your board, you are not doing a good job.

If you are not properly communicating with employers in your community regarding your services and cost of services, you are not doing a good job.

If you are not working closely with your local health systems agency—and I mean in a positive, nonadversary way—you are not doing a good job.

If you have staffed your hospital without regard for efficiency and productivity, you are not doing a good job.

And when you fail to do a good job in all these areas I have mentioned, you are contributing to unnecessary increases in health care costs, to little or no improvement in the quality of care, and to delivering an open invitation to more and more government intervention.

You're already getting far more government help than you want or need in running your hospital. Unless you can find ways to maintain your level of care while containing costs, you're going to get a whole lot more.

Although business generally opposes government regulation and intervention, it knows the critical part that planning plays in any successful and efficient enterprise. Some providers, unhappy with the planning law, have questioned the appropriateness of industry's support, but business, not the provider, pays for the inefficiency and waste that currently exist. Quite appropriately, business seeks to use all available tools to reduce such unnecessary expenditures.

In General Motors, we have urged our management people to become active in the HSA, on boards, on committees, on working groups. Let it be known that we are interested and concerned. I think that the long-range impact might be very favorable.

We have got to do planning or the future is going to be a muddy mirror of the past, and God knows we don't want that. And so with all health planning's faults, our position is that we want to be involved and help it to be as good as it can be.

Victor Zinc

Planning must not be merely a yes or no process. One of the best reasons for business involvement is the technical and financial work that a good HSA must perform if it is to be of use in the community. The HSA in Akron, Ohio, has proven the value of getting tough on such factors as construction costs and interest rates on loans.

> *A hospital goes out and borrows $7 million at an interest rate that isn't competitive on the marketplace. The HSA has already approved the hospital, but if it stops there, it is not doing its job. We call on the private sector, on people who know financing, know investments, and knock off a point [of the interest rate]. Over ten years, this saves the hospital $14 million. Goodyear saves $1.4 million because we are 10 percent of their revenue. That's $1.4 million we can redirect to true health care needs of our employees.*
> Richard Martin

One cannot legitimately separate the interests of providers, consumers, and the community at large. HSAs are a vehicle for bringing all the elements together. Certainly, some will be weakened by fighting among political jurisdictions, some will continue to be dominated by providers, others will be hurt by consumers who fail to make the investment in time that meaningful participation requires. But some are already changing the local delivery system for the common good. More will do so as staffs are developed, the state health plans are completed, and the community as a whole accepts the unavoidable conclusion that local planning is a far better form of rationing than the alternative, which is more federal legislation and regulation.

Industry's support for health planning is not unanimous, but it is growing both in breadth and intensity. Companies such as GENESCO in Tennessee are providing leadership in parts of the country where industry involvement was minimal as recently as early 1977. Several major employers are developing training programs for their officers who serve on the boards of HSAs and hospitals so that they will be equipped to participate on an equal basis with the provider representatives. The WBGH is working to develop a national training resource. The HEW Health Planning Information Center in Atlanta, Georgia, is assisting local HSAs in Region IV to obtain business assistance. The American Health Planning Association is initiating a program to assist and develop the industry-HSA relationship.

The degree of industry support for health planning is directly related to the degree of understanding that industry has come to have of the waste and duplication now driving up their health care costs. Industry's position is reflected in the recent testimony of the WBGH before the Senate Finance Committee. Our recommendations for amendments to P.L. 93–641, the National Health Planning and Resources Development Act, included:

1. A recertification process in certificate of need programs, coupled with strong public disclosure requirements.

2. Decertification and reassignment of a redundant facility's function.

3. The inclusion of all medical and health facilities in certificate of need

calculations (home health, ambulatory care, corporate extended care clinics, leased space, site, and facilities acquisition, and all government beds and facilities).

4. Certification requirements for all large capital expenditures for equipment, no matter where that equipment is to be located.

5. A major effort directed at establishing scientifically valid and publicly accepted measures of health and medical outcomes, cost-benefit relationships, and medical-hospital standards of risk and efficiency.

6. Encouragement, through the certification of need process, of applications with a commitment to good nutrition, immunization, hypertension treatment, and other objectives related to health education and life-style improvement.

7. Retention of the mandatory consumer majority on HSA boards with a commitment of the time and resources necessary to help educate consumer participants who have had little or no prior contact with the health system.

8. Formulation of a national health policy, as called for in P.L. 93–641.

9. Development of a process of medical technology assessment. Its findings should be made available to all health planners and the substance of its deliberations made an ongoing part of medical education. This must be designed to avoid inhibiting innovation and investment in research.[3]

Cooperation vs. Antitrust

We have health planning legislation because Congress and the executive branch have felt pressure from the public to do something to reduce the waste and inefficiencies now so prevalent in our health care delivery system. To achieve this goal, cooperation rather than continued separation and false competition must be encouraged.

The effectiveness of business and labor involvement will frequently depend on the willingness of different companies and unions to share data and combine the economic clout of their work forces. Few, especially outside of headquarters towns, have the concentration of employees to be successful alone.

One result of health planning and the self-initiated efforts to hospitals to contain rising costs has been an increased emphasis upon shared services and facilities. The American Hospital Association reported in July 1977 on the millions of dollars that had been saved by the cooperative efforts of a relatively few hospitals. Is this a positive trend to be encouraged or a dangerous trend to be challenged as a violation of the antitrust laws?

To be effective, health planning, especially before all the states have strong certificate of need programs, must have the cooperation of the financial community. The government has increased its cost containment efforts and reduced the Hill-Burton medical facilities financing program. Therefore, hospital administrators and developers have increasingly turned to the conventional money markets for financing, but local hospital construction financing bonds have become increasingly difficult to sell. The big investors, and there are relatively few despite the rich dollar flow, typically apply a very rigorous return-on-investment analysis before granting the loan. The more responsible among them also ascertain the real need for the proposed facility and cooperate with the HSA. I say *real need* because, with the present reimbursement system, a substantial return on investment can be obtained without regard for need. Were that not so, we would not now be discussing planning and rationing. For the cooperative efforts of the investors to work, all the major funding sources must agree. As Dr. Leon Warshaw has said, "If alternative sources are available, they will be used." And the planning process, at least in the states without effective certificate of need programs, will be circumvented by, for example, the placement of large capital equipment in physicians' offices to avoid rejection in a hospital setting. The use of leased space within the hospital is another example. These actions are possible only if the payer allows charges incurred in such settings to be reimbursed. Another example of the conflict between cooperation and regulation has been a deterrent to insurance industry innovation and progress on cost containment. The economic benefits of competition simply do not exist when the potential for profit is negligible. As a result, the insurance industry has chosen not to provide coverage for those populations who the actuaries have determined could not be covered at a price they can pay. In lieu of protection from the private sector, the government attempts to provide insurance which, in turn, must be financed by increased business, payroll, and personal income taxes. In the past few months, the Senate Antitrust Subcommittee has begun to consider the impact that antitrust regulations have had upon the insurance industry. Senator Kennedy is in the unique position of chairing both this subcommittee and the Health Subcommittee of the Senate Human Resources Committee. No friend of the insurance industry, Senator Kennedy has displayed a new interest in at least examining the possible relaxation of the antitrust regulations to encourage the insurance companies to pool their resources for the benefit of those not now able to afford protection.

In all these situations, our old antitrust policies conflict with our emerging health care cost containment policies. How this conflict is resolved will have a substantial impact on the way industry participates in local health planning. As far as health policy is concerned, much of the traditional labor-management opposition is a myth. In the final analysis, there is only one pot of dollars to be divided among owners, managers, and workers. Health benefits are simply one form of compensation. Labor wants jobs, and industry must have a healthy, stable work force to produce the profits which, when turned into capital investments, return to labor by creating more jobs. Naturally, labor wants to get as large a share of current revenues as possible, while management, just as naturally, is reluctant to part with more than is essential to keep the business operating at a profit.

Health, however, is not something that benefits either labor or management to the exclusion of the other. Waste hurts both equally; for example, unnecessary surgery, or defensive medicine related to fear of malpractice, or stress, or chemical poisoning, or inverted economic incentives that lead to wasted benefits. Setting aside the philosophically different approaches to national health insurance and openly recognizing that some industries have yet to provide even a minimally acceptable level of health benefits, the fact remains that management and labor have common objectives.

Health systems agency boards and committees will increasingly find labor and business sitting together as informed consumers.

HMOs and other alternative delivery systems have the joint support of labor and business.

PSROs and other utilization review groups are finding business and labor jointly insisting on the expansion of concurrent utilization review to all private sector patients.

Business and labor are agreed in their opposition to unnecessary Friday admissions, support for preadmission testing, opposition to wasted technology, support for patients' rights, prospective reimbursement, and health education.

Physicians and hospital administrators find labor and employers jointly supportive of ambulatory care, home health care, prepaid group practices, nutrition counseling, second surgical opinion experiments, appropriate use of physician extenders—and equally concerned about interference in the development of any of these areas.

There are points of congruence for labor and management. Most managements recognize that there is a responsibility for the well-being of their employees.

Melvin Glasser

There needs to be a rededication on the part of management and union people to work together on preventive programs. The law [OSHA] simply says to use the latest available technology. This means the program will be in transition forever.

Glen Wegner

In sum, it is appropriate for labor to press management for improved working conditions and better health benefits. But that should in no way inhibit cooperatively seeking a better health system. Neither labor nor management can reform the health system alone, but together they make a dynamic force for positive change. Together, they—and we—will benefit through reduced waste, abuse, and overutilization. The application of the resulting savings and efficiencies will lead to more equitable distribution of services and access to quality care.

The States' Role

For health planning to work and to warrant increased support from industry, the states must play a major role. Many detractors of the current planning system feel the states are the Achilles heel of the entire system.

> We might try to see social advance [in the health field] in Yale political
> scientist C. E. Lindblom's term *disjointed incrementalism,* in which many
> little pieces move into place with some degree of continuity over time,
> resulting in major and minor improvements. We are never quite as bad as we
> were; we are never quite as good as we are going to be.[4]

This characterizes the role of state government in the health delivery system
today.

Industry finds itself in a quandary about the role of the states in health
policy and regulation. Traditionally and philosophically, industry has supported keeping government intervention at the lowest possible level of political jurisdiction. Therefore, the states appear a more acceptable level than the
federal government for health policy administration. Most of the national
health insurance bills and principles supported by industry include state-level
administration. Yet, the record of the states has been such to cause the leaders
of industry to have second thoughts. For the multistate employer, there are
great complexities and costs associated with meeting the requirements of
national health legislation that is left to the fifty states to administer individually. The growing number of state legislative efforts that conflict with one
another and often with federal legislation is another problem.

Among the big problems in getting the Health Planning and Resources
Development Act implemented have been the slow development of state health
plans, the political fighting between the governors and HEW over HSA area
designation, and the concern that the states would reverse local HSA decisions.
The latter, according to preliminary evaluation, has not been a widespread
problem. But a few instances are resulting in court cases that should ultimately
resolve the jurisdictional issue. So many state health plans are not completed
that Congress is seriously considering a capital expenditure moritorium until
they catch up. Further, approximately 50 percent of the states still do not have
their own certificate of need statutes.

The history of health maintenance organizations provides two other
examples of state-related issues. Problems for the states result from confusion
and conflict between the federal departments of Labor and HEW, concerning
the relationship of HMOs to the pension law (ERISA). The states are left to
interpret that relationship and, in the absence of a uniform federal policy, are
doing so differently. Again, industry feels the cost of extra reporting requirements and is less likely to support HMOs until the confusion is eliminated.

Some states have passed their own HMO laws which differ from the
federal law. For example, in New York, *every* qualified HMO that so requests
must be offered by employers to their employees. The federal law limits the
employer's responsibility to one HMO of each classification (closed-panel or
IPA). In some states, the insurance commissioner is responsible for HMOs, in
California it is the corporation counsel, and other states use other authorities.
All this just makes HMOs less attractive for the multistate employer. Yet, it is
just those employers whom the HMOs must reach if they are to gain enough
enrollment to survive.

Another issue has been the states' failure to resolve the medical malpractice problem. When Congress threatened in 1975 to take federal action to lessen the malpractice liability crisis, the states were adamant that they should be permitted to resolve the problem at their level because of their traditional authority over insurance programs. Two years and an absolute morass of laws later, the problem still exists, the public has seen billions of dollars wasted, the medical profession has resorted to creating its own insurance companies, the federal government is awaiting the results of a major study by the Institute of Medicine, and only one state, California, is conducting a really thorough examination of all relevant aspects of tort law. I might add that the California effort had to be financed by the California Medical Association and other private sources, not the state.

During the endless federal-level national health insurance debate, several states have also passed state health insurance laws. These vary from rather comprehensive programs to those limited to protection from financial catastrophy. All are too new to evaluate (see Exhibit 1). However, they are significant in that if the states do close some of the gaps in insurance coverage, the pressure for NHI will be lessened. In any case, the state programs can serve as experimental models for NHI, and states that do have these new programs will be in a much stronger position either to gain an exemption from NHI or to administer their share of the federal program.

Exhibit 1
State Health Insurance Legislation

State	Type of Legislation[a]	Year Enacted
Rhode Island	Catastrophic	1974
Hawaii	Comprehensive	1974
Connecticut	Comprehensive	1975
Minnesota	Catastrophic	1976
Maine	Catastrophic	1974
Arizona	Catastrophic	1974[b]

[a]Those identified as "catastrophic" are limited to coverage of major medical–type benefits. The "comprehensive" programs include catastrophic coverage as well as a broad spectrum of basic coverage.
[b]Repealed 1976.

States with Health Insurance Bills Currently before the Legislature			
New York	Massachusetts	North Carolina	Oklahoma
Ohio	Kansas	Nebraska	New Mexico
California	Florida	Minnesota	Wisconsin

Sources: There is no single reliable source for state health legislation. These lists were compiled with the assistance of the American Hospital Association and the Health Insurance Association of America.

Exhibit 2
Hospital Prospective Budget and Rate Approval Authorities

Legislation Enacted	Year	Currently before the Legislature
Maryland	1971	California
Massachusetts	1976	Illinois
Connecticut	1973	New Jersey
Washington	1973	Ohio
Colorado	1977	

This list includes only those programs designed to include all patient revenues. A number of other states have more limited programs, but these are generally considered less effective because of the ease with which costs can be shifted to the uncontrolled revenue sources.

Another movement, stimulated specifically by the cost issue, is state rate review authorities. Though small in number, (see Exhibit 2) their impact has already been felt. A hospital cost containment bill now being debated in Congress exempts those states with successful rate review programs from its hospital revenue cap to be federally imposed.

But, how effective will the states be? Their weakness in social service delivery is a result of their own abdication. The "feds" never planned an organized takeover of state functions—the public demanded it. One state took ten years to *start* Medicaid; many are now reducing their share of its financing. Texas is the envy of the world for its high technology (and high publicity) medical centers. The state even had a budget surplus in 1976. Yet, that state fails to provide its thousands of migrant workers with even minimal medical care. Health programs for migrants and seasonal farm workers are primarily federally funded. Because of cases like these and because of media exposure of terrible conditions in some state institutions, many people question the capacity and willingness of the states to do more than pay lip service to the real health delivery problems.

As for many policy problems, the answer seems to lie somewhere between two extremes. The states exist and represent a resource that we as a nation cannot afford to let deteriorate any further. Federal guidelines must be clear, must be enforced, and above all must establish a continuity in service delivery upon which both the server and the served can depend. As we move into the 1980s, the states can play a meaningful role between the neighborhood and the federal government.

Redefining the Industrial Health Program

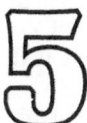

Industry achieved a dubious landmark in 1977: a single company, General Motors, spent more than $1 billion for its employees' health benefits. Despite this vast sum, GM has little influence over the care its premium dollars purchase in many communities. The same is true of most other employers outside their locations of major employment concentration.

Simultaneously, GM and all other manufacturers are being forced to incur great costs and change many operations to comply with four recent laws: the Coal Mine Health and Safety Act (1969), the Occupational Safety and Health Act (1970), the Rehabilitation Act (1973), and the Toxic Substances Control Act (1976). Occupational safety and health regulations are combining with rising costs of health benefits to cause many companies to reexamine their entire approach to the provision of medical and health benefits and services.

> *We discovered that the expectations of our employees coupled with those of society in general were such that a simplistic occupational health program was not sufficient.*
>
> C. Larkin Flanagan et al.

This comment points to one of the major issues facing industry today: is occupational medicine different from nonoccupational? Is there any justification for separating the illness and injury a person may receive at work from all other categories of illness and injury? Currently, industry is divided on whether such a split is justified, but there is general agreement that the distinction is eroding. This is because health and safety regulations and the growing cost escalation problem are driving industry into greater direct provision of care.

Simultaneously, employers are learning that obstacles to a unified care system sometimes emanate from the nonoccupational physicians, some of whom view company programs as an economic threat, especially if the company seeks to establish a closed-panel HMO, and few of whom have a good understanding of the unique characteristics of the work setting, or adequate training in the detection of occupational health problems.

There is also rampant duplication of test results because of the unwillingness of many family physicians and other nonoccupational providers to accept the results of tests done in corporate clinics. The prevalence of extensive insurance and poor claims administration combines with a general skepticism of the quality of industrial medicine to produce this problem.

Some labor leaders also have serious reservations about the quality of industrial medicine as well as concern over its potential use as an instrument of management. They do not welcome an expansion of the role of corporate medical programs. Sheldon W. Samuels of the AFL-CIO expresses it thus:

> The plant situation breeds attitudes inimical to the development of a "normal" physician-patient relationship. . . .
>
> The first and essential view held by workers is that company doctors are no less a part of management than the plant engineer, personnel director, or chairman of the board. They are seen as tools of the boss.[5]

Samuels goes on to highlight the major reasons for this view:

> A company doctor is not legally responsible for malpractice. The company is. . . .
>
> The self-regulation of industrial medicine is much weaker than it is for the other branches of medicine. . . .
>
> The company doctor, even if it is his or her wish, often cannot protect the confidentiality of patient records. . . .
>
> Company medical programs, like any other component of the corporate structure, must justify themselves by dollar benefits. Doctors in this position are less likely to be on the worker's side. . . .
>
> There is general feeling [among workers] that in-plant medical care is of poor quality.[6]

While accepting the fact that all the things Samuels lists are sometimes real problems, many reject the conclusion that industrial medicine should be restricted. There is no reason, the better industrial physicians contend, that an in-house program cannot be as good for the employee-patient as any other medical program. And they resent the inference of being controlled by management. William Greer et al. cite a case at the opposite extreme from Samuels's description:

> At Gillette we tried to transfer private practice into industry. The occupational health physician has the same moral, ethical, and legal obligation to his [or her] employee-patients as to patients in private practice. At Gillette, personal medical records are kept in the medical department and are not subject to review by management.[7]

Despite the reservations of some physicians and some workers, a few companies and some unions have already expanded their medical programs into full service health care delivery systems for all employees and their dependents. Two divergent approaches have been taken by Gillette and R. J. Reynolds (see chapter 7). Gillette built upon a superior industrial medical program to internalize elements of the normal fee-for-service community medical system. Reynolds started from scratch and created a new prepaid HMO as a supplement and competitor to the existing community system.

Another approach, now being explored at the Boston University Health Policy Institute, is a hybrid plan drawing upon the key elements of different programs now in place. The concept was described in a *New England Journal of Medicine* article in June.[8] The group at Boston University hopes to create one or more hybrid demonstrations so the efficacy of the concept can be tested in real conditions. The most attractive aspect of the hybrid is its adaptability to local conditions while preserving the inherent economic advantages of the prepaid, risk-sharing concept.

Whether the idea of expanded medical programs will catch on more generally remains unclear. Their development and their success or failure will be one of the most interesting experiments of the next era of health care delivery. We must recognize, however, that in the near future expanded programs will be implemented by a minority, albeit a very important one, of industry.

The major impetus for expansion, besides the cost of insurance benefits, is the regulation of occupational health and safety by the federal government. However, companies have responded to the laws and regulations in a variety of ways. A spokesman for Monsanto described the company's reaction to the Toxic Substances Control Act thus:

> There was going to be legislation and we thought we'd damn well better get involved to help get legislation and subsequent regulations that are responsible . . . , [otherwise] Congress would have passed a bill more troublesome for both industry and for society, calling for complex testing and duplication of regulation already on the books.[9]

Others did not accept the apparent inevitability of this legislation:

Dow Chemical, however, fought the bill to the end. There were already ample laws on the books to handle any problem that might arise. What's needed is better administration of the laws, not more laws. Kepone was being regulated under the pesticides control and worker safety acts; vinyl chloride under the worker safety and clean air acts.[10]

After OSHA was enacted, it was tied up in court by corporate litigation. Dr. Karl Benedict comments:

Whether or not these legal procedures were intended to nullify the act or any part thereof, they continue and, in truth, have delayed implementation and enforcement of many parts of the act while forcing the secretary responsible for carrying out the intent of Congress to revise administrative procedures, modify enforcement of regulations, conduct prolonged hearings, and delay writing of regulations from criteria documents. Labor has been impatient; industries, confused; and primary care medical clinics have had to mark time or proceed on self-determined courses influenced largely by their own experience.[11]

Dr. Benedict goes on to wonder why some industries are so critical of the functions outlined in the OSHA regulations. "These things should be done to protect the employee first and his fellow worker second. Had they been done voluntarily, OSHA regulations would not have been necessary."[12]

Another corporate reaction to regulation is likely to be a massive increase in the amount and intensity of health screening, or "multiphasic health testing" (MHT), as it is often called. In 1976 the WBGH in conjunction with Arthur D. Little, Inc., conducted a survey of major employers to ascertain the current and anticipated use of MHT. While some firms had used it, either directly or under contract, for years, the survey showed that the primary stimulus to increased use was government regulation, specifically OSHA. Companies simply have no choice under the safety laws but to screen their exposed employees—and frequently even job applicants. Without the data base thereby developed, there is no way to measure the impact of future exposure to pollutants and toxic substances.

Currently, most companies that have screening programs seem to feel they are valuable in themselves, aside from the part they play in complying with regulations. Most feel that such programs ought to include a schedule based on age, sex, job category, and prior medical history of the worker to be tested.

Gillette's evaluation of their MHT program is illustrative:

The health survey is not designed primarily with the aim of making startling discoveries of serious physical impairment, even though defects, both major and minor, will be found. On the average, only about 65 percent of any population seems to have "preferred" or standard health profiles, meaning that they are free of minor or major defects. The benefits of the health survey are that it:

Preserves good health. This is the primary objective.

Makes people health conscious. It is important to know that you are well. Minor conditions or complaints are often borne in silence as one of the routine burdens inherent in the process of living.

Overcomes fear of examination. Some people dread examination because something seriously wrong might be found. If the examination is normal, then considerable apprehension may be relieved.

Banishes false disease symptoms. Some fear disease to such an extent that they may actually experience symptoms of the disease that they secretly believe they have, the most common being heart disease. Dispelling false fears is excellent treatment for getting back into a normal healthy state of mind.

Reveals physical defects. This is not the total motivation for health surveys, but serious problems may be discovered early enough for remedial treatment. Correction or treatment of potentially serious problems discovered may avert later, more serious or chronic conditions or complications.

Reveals causes other than physical defects for poor health, such as poor living habits or emotional problems.

Gives an opportunity for teaching good health habits.[13]

In addition to MHT, some companies have chosen to use other screening procedures such as pap smears and glaucoma tests. However, employers are in a quandary when trying to measure the cost-effectiveness of such procedures. Both advocates and critics abound. Considered individually, the procedures are not expensive and their payoff, both emotional and financial, can be considerable.

> *For every case of glaucoma I can find in Boise Cascade employees, I can save the corporation $15,000.*
>
> Glen Wegner

On the other hand, the cost may be small per person but very high per positive outcome. New York Telephone has 40,000 female employees. According to Dr. Collings:

If I do a pap smear once a year as a good clinician would recommend, and if I do it as cheaply as anybody has ever done them, with follow-up, that's about $10, so we have $500,000 per year invested. From that population, I get two cases of cervical cancer per year.

Each cancer discovery costs the company $250,000.

Finally, federal regulations have had the effect of changing the basic nature of many companies' screening programs.

The format of the medical program in my company has changed from comprehensive, general medical examinations and limited treatments to more frequent, limited, yet more intense studies of certain persons in jobs identified by OSHA in new regulations. New laboratory procedures in-plant or outside will be required as new chemicals and related regulations are developed . . . There will be increased costs in equipment, record keeping, and personnel.[15]

Successful screening does not mean the end of corporate responsibility, however:

> We have uncovered a whole Pandora's box of medical problems through the screening required by the new coke oven emission standards. It's scary and exciting at the same time: scary, because there is no health care system to turn these facts over to and say "you guys follow up on these coincidential findings"; but exciting because it opens up the possibility of a whole new type of health care delivery that may have to be sparked by industry.
>
> Joseph Miller

Increased responsibilities face the employer because a certain percentage of people tested are bound to evidence serious health problems. The problems uncovered may have nothing to do with the purpose of the test, but once they are found, there is a moral and perhaps legal obligation to follow up with information, referral, or even treatment.

One of the difficulties industry faces when trying to implement the new regulations is their not infrequent conflict with other regulations. For example, preemployment testing will become increasingly stringent to meet the requirements that people's susceptibility to various chemicals and pollutants be measured. However, Equal Employment Opportunity and Federal Employment of the Handicapped programs may well file suit against the employer who uses a potential health risk as the justification for employment rejection.

Similar issues arise when health tests are given to existing employees. The medical department's split responsibility between the patient and the company is further complicated by a responsibility to the full community of employees and the community at large. To further complicate matters, employees are understandably divided in their desires to continue working and to avoid additional exposure to some harmful chemical. However, the company is responsible for informing employees of the problem and protecting them from further exposure.

The whole question of a company's post-screening responsibilities combines with the difficulty of measuring screening's cost-effectiveness to make many companies reluctant to proceed. Some costs can be measured if the hidden expenses inherent in certain policy decisions can be identified. Greer et al. noted that it costs Gillette $25,000–30,000 to train one machinist; thus, even a $15,000 medical expense may be a saving to the company if it enables it to retain a trained machinist. Similarly, Gillette pays opthalmologists high fees to come to the plant rather than sending the employees out for glaucoma tests. The reason:

> If the employee goes outside, you know it takes less than an hour

to actually see the doctor. But he [the employee] takes about five hours stopping for lunch, missing the subway, having coffee, etc. We feel we save money by paying the doctor extra to come to the employee.

William E. Greer

Some, however, would prefer to ignore the cost-effectiveness issue entirely, feeling it is not an appropriate concern for industrial physicians:

I would protest the search for cost-effectiveness per se for any given technique, procedure, or device. It depends on how you use it, where you use it, and whether it was needed. I think our job as professionals is to look at the resources we've got and not fall into the trap of immediately trying to judge whether something is cost-effective.

G. H. Collings

But cost-effectiveness is an inevitable concern in a resource-limited, demand-unlimited situation. Its measures are a basic tool for reasoned priority-setting. Unfortunately for the corporate physician or policymaker, even the so-called superstars of the medical world are unable, at this point, to resolve the dilemma.

The coronary bypass operation is often cited as a perfect example of the problem. If everyone who wanted the operation were to receive it at current rates, a multibillion dollar allocation to this one procedure would result. This is the cost-effectiveness issue on a grand scale. Dr. Denton Cooley, the premier practitioner and advocate of this technique, speaks for one side:

There are a million new candidates for coronary bypass surgery each year. Right now we operate on fifty thousand of them, which means nine hundred and fifty thousand aren't getting helped. My feeling is we should try to help everyone we can.[16]

Dr. Cooley himself conducts some 1,500 bypass operations each year in addition to more than 1,000 other heart operations. His views are opposed by Dr. John Norman, also a heart surgeon:

I just don't think an expensive operation is the answer to this problem. What you want is something like penicillin that costs seven cents. If you need an iron lung, special hospitals, and special doctors to cure polio, you don't really have a cure. The world really doesn't need a hundred more Doctor Cooleys. Most of the expensive cures like open-heart surgery aren't really cures. They are palliatives. What we are doing today is probably obsolescent and in a short span of time will become antediluvian.[17]

Regardless of cost, people will line up to be saved by Dr. Cooley until that penicillin injection is available. And one thing is certain: industry pays much of the bill and has no voice in the decision.

One of the few reasons cost-effectiveness analysis is so difficult is that there are few publicly known and accepted standards by which medical outcomes can be measured. Nor has industry collected the data to adequately access what it pays for in the health care area. The few companies such as Goodyear and Ford that have made the investment in data collection and analysis show its value. Industry will be the loser unless it has the data to support its positions in cost containment negotiations. But primarily, data are crucial to the establishment and enforcement of professional standards.

The idea of medical standards has always evoked images of Big Brother and of mechanical, dehumanized treatment. However, a little known fact is that some 800 medical societies, specialty boards, and government authorities *already* promulgate medical diagnosis and treatment standards. Let us be clear about what standards are and what problems surround them:

They are a guide, a starting point, a minimum acceptable performance.

They should never be static. As new knowledge is gained and new technology developed, the standards must be adapted.

They are not value judgments, but should be based on objective criteria.

They are currently a morass of duplication, conflict, and contradiction, as anything emanating from so many sources is found to be.

They are frequently ignored by the providers simply through ignorance of their existance.

They are virtually unknown and unavailable to the medical care purchaser and consumer.

They will be of growing importance to industry as its role as provider expands, as scrutiny of the returns on industry's health expenditures increase, and as peer review programs include more and more private patients and ambulatory patients.

The major standards effort in recent years has been the government's Professional Standards Review Organization (PSRO) program. Based on the concepts of peer and utilization review and building on the private sector foundations for medical care programs, the PSRO legislation is an attempt by Congress to give the medical profession the opportunity to regulate itself.

Industry representatives who have examined the PSRO effort feel it has been marginally effective—in some places excellent, but in most weak and restricted to patients whose care is publicly financed. Nonetheless, certain characteristics of PSRO review make it an attractive concept for industry:

It is conducted at the most local of levels, the hospital.

It is done *by* physicians rather than *to* them.

If well done, this makes the physician an ally of cost containment, without placing industry in the uncomfortable position of seeming to tell the physician how to practice.

It is basically a private sector program.

It generates data that are needed for planning.

To quote Dr. Himler, "The mere knowledge that a review system is operative has a salutary deterrent effect on individuals [physicians] who are habitually abusers."[18]

However, the detractors of PSRO abound. For instance, Henry Damm says:

> PSROs are using very general guidelines that have not been documented from a medical-scientific or medical-legal standpoint. They are, in short, a throwback to the outdated community standard of practice and are counter-productive to any national cost and quality control effort.[19]

One does not have to be so harsh to note that PSROs are indeed beset by serious problems. By dealing almost exclusively with public sector patients, they limit their impact because cost shifting can replace cost saving. Also, their objectivity is called into question by some on the grounds of their close connection with the medical profession. One of their strengths—their being local—is also one of their weaknesses since it perpetuates the wide and totally unnecessary regional variations in cost and length-of-stay standards for identical procedures. There is no medical justification for these variations, and no need for each community to develop its own standards. Finally, PSROs are less than adequate in scope because they do not review the two most rapidly expanding areas of medical care: ambulatory and home care.

Henry Damm believes that an orderly, accurate, and rather low-cost system for improving professional standards review already exists. He is working with large employers to redirect their purchasing power toward improved medical outcomes.

> The purchasers of health services must have valid data on an ongoing basis to be able to measure the services received, that is to know whether they are getting the best value for the dollar. They must be able to measure the effects of any cost control approach to know in advance what the trade-offs will be with the quality of outcomes. Outcomes can be measured statistically and actuarially by the spillover effect of health services on sick pay, disability benefits, workers' compensation, death benefits, absenteeism, cost of retraining, and cost of rehabilitation.[20]

Damm has been working for the past year with a group of employers (TRW, AT&T, Sun Co., Uniroyal, Dayco, Sears) to develop a data system that will guide purchasers in designing and administering benefits less conducive to wasteful utilization by their employees.

In short, a system with uniform standard criteria is needed to assure that only those services will be used that result in the least amount of preventable death or disease, and provide the best outcome with the least cost, and that those services will be given in both the medical and spillover areas.[21]

Standards and data are also a vital element of increasing the capacity of the consumer to understand alternatives and make wise choices. Rarely does the patient-consumer-purchaser of medical services have the benefit of comparative information on cost or quality of care. Physicians and medical facility administrators have understandably been loath to make such information available.

With or without standards or cost-benefit analysis or any other measure of the value of medical procedures or of detection and prevention programs, industry must face the biggest challenge on its own: what to do with the workers in whom are detected previously undiagnosed illnesses or who are shown to be susceptible to injury or whose profiles indicate that continuation in their present jobs could endanger their health. This dilemma and the others highlighted above produce what Equitable's Dr. Leon Warshaw calls "the schizoid situations in which we find ourselves."

Industrial Health Programs: Dimensions and Issues

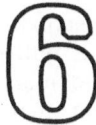

Federal regulations and concern over the growing cost of health insurance benefits have combined to impel many companies to redefine and expand the responsibilities of the corporate medical department. This is no simple task. There are a number of dimensions of possible redefinition and a number of issues that a company must face in becoming more fully a health care provider. The health care needs of a changing work force complicate the provision of health care. The spectre of health-related liability grows as corporate health services expand. Finally, two areas little known in previous industrial health programs present themselves for possible inclusion in a program designed to improve the health status of the work force while minimizing the cost of health services. These are health education and mental health services or benefits.

Our Changing Work Force

The typical profile of the American worker is a white male who works for one company all his life while his wife stays home with three or more children. With his family he takes two weeks' vacation every year and looks forward to retirement at a predetermined age. At least seven major trends are now at work reshaping that profile. Any health policy or industry benefit strategy must recognize these changes and consider their impact on the health-related needs of the American worker.

The first is the growing number of women in the work force. The men may not be going into the kitchen but the women are definitely going to work, and this movement is not likely to be reversed. The impacts are immediate (the pregnancy disability issue) and complex (toxic substances exposure impacts on the reproductive process). There will also be pressure for day care benefits as more families have both parents working. The second trend is toward fewer children in the American family. The smaller family means a changed benefit package with fewer dependents to cover and different demands for services upon which experience ratings will be calculated. Third, mandatory retirement age levels have been dropping. Now, it appears they may be eliminated entirely or modified by federal and/or state legislation, as was passed in California in September 1977. Concerned that mandatory retirement discriminates against the fastest growing segment of the population, Congress is likely soon to either extend the retirement age or prohibit it entirely. Of course, this will not be welcomed by those seeking to advance or to gain entry-level employment. And, it will certainly have an impact on the type of medical benefits that are utilized, as well as on the intensity of their use. The relaxation of mandatory retirement will increase the average age of the work force, as will the fourth trend: the increase in the median age of the population. The elderly are a rapidly growing percentage of the population, both because people are living somewhat longer and, more importantly, because today's young families are having fewer children. From the standpoint of utilization of medical resources, this is probably the single most important trend.

Equal opportunity laws have recently been expanded to include handicapped persons. And, as more ethnic minorities become college graduates, it will be increasingly difficult to refuse them employment through the old subterfuge of "unqualified." The design and utilization of medical programs and benefits will have to reflect the physical and cultural needs of these new employment groups.

For Congress and the administration, unemployment is of course a much larger political and economic problem than national health insurance. Government work programs and/or incentives for the private sector to hire more of the unemployed, especially the young, is one type of response. Another is the recently announced welfare program, which will have a work requirement and a redesigned payment schedule intended to reverse the disincentives the current program has for either working or for maintaining a nuclear family. Both these programs are long-range efforts aimed at decreasing dependency by increasing individual purchasing capacity.

The impact that these six trends will have on health and medical care will not always be measurable but the seventh, increased leisure time, is likely to be the most significant. Injuries and illness incurred during time off are just as costly to the employer but far harder for the employer to prevent than those incurred at work. If we accept the contention that our life-style is the single largest determinent of our health status, then major changes in the proportion of time spent not working will have an impact on health and health costs.

An alternative result of more leisure time is not necessarily more leisure at all. Many find, for either financial or emotional reasons, that a second job is more attractive than longer hours in front of the television set. The industry health policy implications of this development are extremely complex. Which employer provides what benefits? Who pays if an employee incurs a medical expense while on vacation from both jobs? Which policy covers dependents? When one employer offers coverage for dentistry and the other for vision care, what controls the employee's selection and what are the implications for utilization, for switching at open enrollment times, and so on? A related issue is the decrease of a single-career lifestyle. Many more people are changing careers at points and with a frequency unheard of only ten years ago. This raises issues of the portability of health insurance and the lack of uniformity among programs.

Taken together, these changes will have a dramatic impact on all of us, on our life-style, our standards of living, and, unavoidably, on the role of the employer in health care. As all these changes take place, they add to the liability burden facing employers in a litigation-happy era.

The New Issue of Liability

As if the pressures of product liability were not enough, corporations delivering medical and health care must now be concerned with an array of new liability issues. Corporate medical departments must carry malpractice insurance, a fact that has caused some critics to accuse industrial physicians of being less prudent than their self-employed counterparts who purchase their own malpractice protection. Their defenders content that the pressures of employment provide industrial physicians with strong incentives to do the best possible job. From a policy perspective, the intriguing question is to what degree the existence of—and uncertainty about—liability causes industry to move reluctantly into the direct provision and management of health and medical care.

OSHA and the Toxic Substances Control Act are rapidly forcing the employer into the role of health status analyst, monitor, and, in effect, guardian. There are as yet too few legal cases for employers to know the extent of their liability. The extent of the potential problem, however, is obvious considering that the Toxic Substances Control Act alone will require over 20 million workers to be screened at least annually. The number of medical problems discovered, quite apart from those the tests were designed to identify, will be staggering and will give rise to numerous questions of responsibility for follow-up, payment, confidentiality, and so forth.

With so much uncertainty, it is not surprising that many major employers simply assume they are liable for medical malpractice and insure themselves accordingly. This can be a devastating expense, especially for smaller employers, and often an unanticipated one, apparently unrelated to their medical care performance record.

> *One of the most appalling business experiences I ever went through was renegotiating our malpractice insurance. After eighteen years and never having had a malpractice claim, our insurance carrier wanted to increase our premiums tenfold.*
>
>   Stanley deLisser

The liability issue affects industry because as John Blum says, "once the employer comes to the assistance of the employee, that assistance must be provided with appropriate care under the general principles of tort law."[22] A relatively large number of cases can be expected because recent media coverage of major occupational health problems has brought liability issues to the attention of the public, of lawyers, and of employees.

Many work-related injuries and illnesses are covered by state workers' compensation laws, but there is little uniformity in their administration and great disparity in their judicial interpretations. The expansion of workers' compensation to include aggravation of preexisting nonoccupational illness and injury will add to the confusion as the Toxic Substances Control Act is fully implemented.

The dividing line between a work-related and non-work-related injury or illness is often very vague and judgmental, yet it is of vital concern from the liability standpoint. The precedents for liability in cases of injury or illness not covered by workers' compensation are even more uncertain than for those covered. Historically, the company was responsible only to hire qualified physicians. Today,

> the company incurs liability for the negligent conduct of physicians it employs. The duty of the corporation to hire competent medical personnel includes a responsibility not to retain the services of a physician who becomes unfit or incompetent over time.
>
> The corporation's duty to ensure that physicians who deliver medical care under corporate auspices maintain a continuing competence requires some type of monitoring of physician behavior. The role of the corporation as a monitor of the medical services it provides for its employees may in fact be significantly extended with an increase in corporate clinic services. The company that provides medical services for its employees directly is producing health care as one of its products and, in fact, takes on a role analogous to other health care institutions.[23]

The employer is liable not only through the doctrine of respondeat superior (making it responsible for the actions of its agents), but also liable should there be any gains from providing health services, which makes the company legally a medical provider. Unfortunately, there is no common defi- nition of what constitutes an employer's "gain." Blum cites the Ohio Supreme Court in *Procter v. Ford Motor Company:*

> The business of Ford is manufacturing automobiles; yet to say that its maintenance of a full-staffed plant medical facility is unrelated to produc- ing cars ignores the reality of modern industrial life. Ford's business inter- est in efficiency of operation is directly served by providing readily accessi- ble medical care to those workmen whose minor injuries or ailments might otherwise result in their absence from the production line. . . . So while there is no doubt that the workmen are most directly served by a plant dispensary, it is equally clear that appellant physicians are employed in work that furthers the business interests of their employer.[24]

There can be little doubt that the issue of malpractice liability is having an impact on decisions to expand corporate medical facilities and programs. Even in health education there lurks the spectre of a suit based on a negative outcome when corporate, or just corporately distributed, advice is followed. Even more uncertain is whether there is liability for not disseminating certain types of information. For large companies, these problems, although signifi- cant, will not prohibit providing health care. For smaller ones, the cost of malpractice insurance alone is a major barrier to the direct provision of medical care.

Toward the other end of the spectrum of corporate concerns for liability is the issue of health education. In rhetoric, health education is linked more to motherhood and apple pie than to the meaningful reform of the health system. Yet it may be, and many in industry are increasingly taking this position, that health education is the single most important element of that reform.

Health Education

Few areas in the whole health field are as little understood or as poorly funded as health education, but few have so much potential to reduce unneces- sary utilization and to improve the health status of our population. There is no definitive budget analysis to show what portion of the $139.4 billion we spent for health care in 1976 went for health education, but authorities like John Knowles, Lester Breslow and Anne Somers all agree that it does not exceed 1 percent.

Yet nearly everyone connected with health agrees that the public and the medical profession are in need of a large injection of health education. One indication is that the public demand for medical care bears little relation to actual need. In fact, many physicians and medical authorities believe that between 33 and 66 percent of all visits to primary care physicians are medically unnecessary. Demand must be modified, especially if we move to a national health insurance system. Regardless of what system or formula we select to guide our rationing of medical resources, education of the provider, the patient, and general public will be essential.

For providers, today's education must supply what yesterday's left undone: patient communication skills, cost-conscious selection of treatment modalities, prevention, patients' rights, and so forth. Patients, too, need education about their rights and options while under treatment. Perhaps most important, our school system simply must include health education at all levels. Physical education and occasional sex education are provided but touch only two of the many areas that should be ongoing parts of curricula. Even the legislated health programs such as immunization frequently fail to reach a large percentage of their target groups and nutrition is left to the corner candy store. Rarely does a school work with the families on a total approach to health education.

The escalation of medical care costs has led to the realization that all of us must become more responsible for our own health and less dependent on a medical care system that simply cannot satisfy all our demands. This means we must make healthful modifications in our life-styles—stop smoking, eat less and better food, get more exercise, and so on (see Exhibit 3). Cost escalation has also led to the growing effort among large health insurance purchasers to educate their employees on the appropriate use of their benefits. It is true that our poorly designed, very comprehensive insurance packages are a major stimulus to cost increases. But it is equally true that consumers can be trained to use those benefits wisely, for the sake of their health if not their finances. "Overutilization is bad for your health" may become the watchword of health benefit administrators.

Individual employers spend millions on pay envelope enclosures, video presentations, and time off for lectures or specialized clinics. Yet little evaluation is performed, follow up is weak, and most companies start their own programs with little regard to the successes or failures of others. However, the commitment to education is growing. Industry has been a principal force behind the creation of the National Center for Health Education. Serious consideration is being given to the development of a special center for information exchange and analysis of corporate-based health education programs.

But many inconsistencies remain. Tobacco companies teach the evils of alcohol, while liquor manufacturers hold stop-smoking clinics. Innoculations are provided free if foreign travel is on business but not for vacation, despite the obvious fact that disease-caused lost time is just as costly no matter what the origin of the trip. Few benefit programs contain incentives to monitor, let alone change, life-styles. Employers do not wish to be seen as dictating behavior. Yet, they do want to stop paying for the health damage caused by poor behavior, behavior often stemming from ignorance of its consequences to health.

Health education is a boundless field, an objective probably never to be fully achieved, but it has great potential for improving human lives while reducing the rate at which we are presently wasting our limited resources. The time to begin is now and industry can play a major role. Many companies are

Exhibit 3
The Association of Behavior and Ill Health

Disease & Other Conditions \ Behavior	Accident Proneness	Alcohol Abuse	Poor Childbearing Practices	Inadequate Parenting	Cigarette Smoking	Inappropriate Diet	Insufficient Exercise	Excessive Stress
Accidents	X	X						
Arthritis								X
Asthma								X
Bone & Joint Problems	X							
Bronchitis & Emphysema					X			
Cerebrovascular Disease					X	X	X	
Child Abuse				X				
Cirrhosis of the Liver		X				X		X
Diabetes						X	X	
Heart Disease					X	X	X	X
Homicide		X		X				X
Hypertension						X	X	X
Infant Mortality			X		X			
Malignant Neoplasms		X			X	X	X	
Mental & Nervous Conditions		X		X				X
Spinal Cord Injury	X							
Peptic Ulcer					X	X		X
Suicide		X		X				X
Wounds & Lacerations	X	X						

Source: Rhode Island Department of Health, *Health Behavior Intervention in Rhode Island*, Providence, R.I., September 1976.

already doing something; a few are doing a lot and are making real innovations that may be transferable to other settings.

A commitment to health education carries with it a commitment to learn the real needs of the employees. Mobil Oil is an example:

> *The part-time psychiatrist we have at our headquarters is there not only to treat people. He is there to examine the corporation and how they treat people.*
>
> H. A. Sinclaire

Dr. Sinclaire noted that this commitment resulted in a study of the impact a change of management had on the employees: "We saw a tremendous increase in hypertension, with anxiety depression and peptic ulcer disease."[25] Mobil is also cooperating with the Norwegian government to study the health risk factors of those living on the North Sea oil platforms. "There are lots of things we feel we can prevent by teaching management better ways of handling people and by studying on-platform safety mechanisms to make people feel more at home."[26]

Alcoa has expanded their definition of health education to include training for corporate officers who serve on hospital boards.

> For many years Alcoans have served on boards of hospitals in the communities in which we are located.
>
> [Early in March] we surveyed 16 locations where we have plants and found that 19 Alcoans are serving with hospitals boards, 15 as board members, and 4 as presidents of the hospital board.
>
> In two of these locations there is an interesting story to tell:
>
> > At one West Coast location the manager of our plant was the key to consolidation of two community hospitals. Over a four-year period the manager in addition to attending the board meetings of the hospital, attended more than 50 meetings, some of which involved trips to communities as far as 100 miles away, to learn from experience in those communities.
> >
> > It is estimated that this consolidation will save the community $325,-000 a year and will have a significant reduction in capital improvement without sacrificing the quality of care. Our manager was joined by representatives of several other companies in helping make this consolidation possible.
> >
> > At another location in the Midwest the manager of our facility has been working for over 5 years to accomplish a merger of two community hospitals. The merger was undertaken when one of the two hospitals proposed to the Community Health Planning Agency at $12 million expenditure. The Community Health Planning Agency turned down the request. It was appealed to the State and Regional offices and turned down by both offices. The agency did recommend merger discussions.

The manager was chairman of a task force which undertook the study to consolidate. The activities of our manager along with other industrial and civic leaders in the community have resulted in Articles of Incorporation approved by both boards and a total of 18 other points for consolidation.

Recognizing the importance of having responsible people serve on hospital boards we have developed a hospital trustee training program which will be used to train all Alcoa employees appointed to hospital boards who wish to use it.[27]

Alcoa has also recognized the need to extend their safety program beyond the traditional in-plant bounds.

We studied off-the-job injuries at one plant. We found that in one year 111 employees were injured, 4 of them fatally. We estimated a total cost of $340,000 for that year—NOT including survivors' benefits or many of the indirect expenses which arise when an employee is injured. Working with the safety department, we propose to set up more off-the-job safety programs on subjects such as: defensive driving, camping, power tools, boating, snowmobiling, bicycling, skiing, firearms, home safety.[28]

Another example is Continental Bank which has recently initiated a new health education program which goes way beyond the more traditional methods of information dissemination:

We propose to help employees become better health care consumers by educating them at the time they plan to make use of major health services. It is our feeling that the employee/patient today does not have the necessary information on which to base a rational consumer decision. The patient often follows the doctor's fatherly advice without question as to the necessity for recommended medical or surgical treatment. Many patients consider it to be "bad form" to ask the doctor about his fees. The doctor in this case is viewed as a lifesaver. Putting a dollar value on life is impossible, especially when it is your own.

Effective May 1, 1977 our personnel employee benefit health insurance claim administrators will begin to consult with employees before a hospital stay. Through an experimental second opinion for elective surgery program with Chicago Blue Cross–Blue Shield, the patient will be able to assess the necessity of recommended treatment. Employees who wish a second opinion will be given a list of three certified specialists whom they can consult with or without their doctor's knowledge to obtain a second or even a third opinion on the course of treatment recommended.

Our Blue Shield insurance plan covers 80 percent of usual and customary doctors' charges. When a doctor charges more than usual and customary, the patient pays 100 percent of the excess. Today when this happens, it is a surprise to the patient. After the care has been rendered he or she finds out from Blue Shield that a portion of the bill is not covered.

Effective May 1, we will be able to provide information about the impact of usual and customary charge limits to employees who have obtained detailed price and treatment information from their physician before treatment is rendered. An employee who asks his or her doctor to write down his fee and the procedure he plans to use, using medical terminology, can come to our employee benefit office and find out beforehand if part of that fee will be beyond usual and customary limits. This, then, will provide him information with which to judge the doctor's price and eliminate the useless surprise when it is too late to do anything. This "predetermination of benefit" is being done as a joint experiment by Blue Cross–Blue Shield and Continental Bank.[29]

Implicit in this discussion of health education is a willingness on the part of industry to explore new approaches to cost containment, to accept a broader definition of their health responsibilities, and to recognize that the barriers between occupational and nonoccupational health are reduced if not removed.

These same forward-looking, although admittedly neither universally accepted nor widely implemented concepts are being applied to the health issue which I feel may prove to be the most critical for the remainder of this century: mental health.

Mental Health

We really are a quite healthy society, and we should be spending more time and energy acknowledging this, and perhaps trying to understand why it is so. We are in some danger of becoming a nation of healthy hypochondriacs.[30]

Lewis Thomas

Hypochondriacs cost us all a lot of money. Or, as Dr. John Knowles put it, "one man's freedom in health is another man's shackle in taxes and insurance premiums."[31] Each year, millions of physician visits and an appreciable number of hospital stays are purchased for no discernible medical reason. "Kaiser-Permanente, in a study of 1,250,000 subscribers, found that 68 percent of the people who came for treatment had no organic cause for their complaint."[32] A major portion of this cost is borne by insurance companies; many analysts believe the consumer might act differently if the money for all this nonmedical care had to be paid out of pocket. Perhaps so, but even more basic questions must be asked. What is driving all these people to feel that they need medical care? What can we offer in place of the physician to provide a legitimate source of relief for the "patient"? And, what role is there for industry in this process of social change?

The answers to these questions may be found in a combination of what can be loosely described as health education and mental health care. Through the years, our health system has done little—and has provided few incentives—to encourage the public not to use its services. Our educational system perpetuated the myth that physicians were the only ones who could understand, let alone repair, the human body, and little has yet to enter curricula at any level to help people gain greater understanding and responsibility for their health. Today, policymakers, with one eye on rising medical care costs, are calling on us to assume a greater role in our own care. In theory, this is very reasonable and, in the long run, necessary. In reality, this is a pipe dream unless the educational system develops the capacity to give us this new awareness. It is fine to tell the consumer to challenge the physician, but the effort is sure to be wasted unless there are alternative avenues to information and, when necessary, treatment.

Not surprisingly, it has been cost more than concern that has opened the door. More and more, the linkages between psychological problems and physical medicine overutilization have become apparent, and medical treatment is frequently more expensive and less satisfactory to the patient than the early and proper treatment of the emotional problem.

Mental health benefits can, however, serve to contain medical overutilization. The Kaiser study noted that "when a mental health program was added as an intervention plan, medical utilization over a five-year period was reduced by 60 percent by those attending a *single* psychotherapy session."[33] In California there is a new prepaid mental health program called the California Psychological Health Plan, whose aggressive educational effort and phased-in benefit structure assures the patient needed care while guarding against overutilization. The results in a first-year test group show a 20 percent reduction in the use of medical care benefits. The concept is simple and best described by its designer, John Armer:

> We have a closely monitored panel of providers who work in their own private offices throughout the State. We have tried to overcome the problems dealing with delivering mental health services. *First:* No cost (no deductible, no copayments) for the first five visits—we encourage utilization. *Second:* Easy access to providers—the subscriber is told (and shown) that providers are available wherever they need them "close to home or work." *Third:* Confidentiality—in my opinion, this is the greatest need of all in this somewhat difficult area of health care. There are no claim forms. We tell subscriber employees, that no one in the office and no one at home, if you don't want to discuss the problem right now, needs to know. *Fourth:* Quality control—we are using paid providers who have agreed to several major requirements: They must attend professional standards and management meetings—in-service training, continuing education (in fact, we have arranged continuing education credit for these sessions), which are held in major population centers throughout the state. The providers agree to our usual, customary, and regular fee. They also must agree to our reserving 20 percent of this fee—necessary now while we are learning more about utilization, and—this is the really important one—we tell subscribers they don't have to worry about getting slipshod advice or walking into the wrong office.

> Our providers must agree to professional standards and management meetings before they proceed with their consultation beyond the fifth visit. If the subscriber and provider agree it is a good idea to go beyond the fifth visit,

the provider must appear before a local panel of his or her colleagues to discuss the case in question. Again, confidentiality is complete. No names or identification are used. The case is discussed with respect to diagnosis, prognosis, and treatment plan—the old-fashioned "peer review" system is a thing of the past. This is a cooperative, collaborative, educational meeting with groups of professionals lending their best expertise to a system of health care—they are attempting to serve our subscribers in the best way possible.

Industry's record in providing mental health benefits, though much stronger than many presume, is still not sufficient. Prepayment is rare. So too is pressure on the insurance carriers to design innovative programs.

Industry holds the key to making substantial progress in the mental health arena because it is safe to say that unless these services are offered as a covered benefit, they will not be an available, affordable option for most people. But, just providing the insurance is not enough: the educational component is essential.

The WBGH conducted a survey in June 1977, of mental health programs of 145 major employers. The data in the 79 replies supports the theory that industry is and must be a major force for the integration of mental and physical health benefits. All 79 companies have a mental health program, although most offer a mental health insurance benefit rather than direct care. Most of the responding companies stated that they now consider mental illness just another disease and do not maintain separate cost and utilization data for these benefits. This hampers evaluation but it is a sign of significant progress in attitudes toward mental illness and its treatment. Some problems (alcoholism, depressive disorders) are very commonly covered, while others (family and sexual problems) are just starting to be accepted. There is a sharp distinction within the mental health benefits programs between the more well-known and visible illnesses and those that are perhaps more common but have yet to receive the public and media attention that appears necessary to make them acceptable for coverage.

Mental health benefit programs tend to have more cost-sharing than the physical health programs, and have been designed with more awareness of the reimbursement mechanism's power to guide utilization. Outpatient care is regularly covered, as is nonhospital inpatient care. Many programs (65 percent) allow reimbursement for "in-residence" programs which allow the patient to spend some time at work or home, as professionally appropriate. Nonphysician practitioners' services are regularly 80 percent covered.

Of the 79 replies, between 46 and 53 percent reported the following encouraging results: lower employee absenteeism, improved productivity, improved employee morale, fewer instances of reported severe mental illness (leading to the conclusion that a prevention program can have positive results), and reduced hospital utilization.

However, despite the growing evidence of the savings, in both dollars and suffering, that result from an affirmative mental health program, few of even the most progressive companies devote more than a minor share (5 percent on the average) of their total health benefits funds to this category. Many companies are expanding their programs, but there is little indication of major innovation or pressure from industry on the insurance and provider communities to provide the emphasis on mental health that is needed.

The results of our survey are certainly positive and should be enough to support the expansion of industry programs, but problems do remain. Despite the reduction in severe cases and the reduction in hospital utilization, only 16 percent of the respondents could report a reduction in their insurance premiums. And the two most frequently cited barriers to the development and use of a mental health program were "identifying employees in need of assistance" and "removing stigmas associated with treatment of mental health." Even in the alcoholism programs, progress is far from satisfactory. It is easy to view the efforts of the leading, very large employers and forget that they are not representative of employers generally. "Companies are neglecting the consequences of alcoholism because alcoholism is still considered a self-inflicted moral problem. . . . Also, alcoholics can conceal their illness until it is in its terminal stages. And, alcohol is an accepted social and business lubricant. [Considering that] alcoholic workers cost American corporations at least $15 billion annually in absenteeism, poor judgment, decreased productivity, accidents, disguised hospital and medical claims"[35] it would seem reasonable that all companies work to build solutions into their personnel policies and benefit programs. In the decade ahead, the contribution of mental health benefits to cost savings should give industry the necessary incentive to take a leadership role on this difficult issue. The opportunities here for self-interest and public interest to merge are too significant to ignore.

Models of Industry Involvement

Medical care costs, increased appreciation of the complexity of our total health care system, perceptions of grossly wasted resources, and growing—and conflicting—government regulations have all combined to create industry's desire to gain more direct control over its health care investment. As the few corporate leaders who have become publicly known for their innovative efforts can attest, there is a voracious appetite among employers for models that could lead to cost-effective improvements in health and medical care programs. Several models already exist and they are showing the way to the ideal combination of better quality care and a reduced rate of cost escalation. Further, they are the pragmatic manifestations of the changing role of industry in health care.

Commonalities and Caveats

Before describing the specific models, it may be useful to point out what they have in common. This is especially important in light of the primary caveat: they were not designed to be models and thus make no claim to be replicable without significant modification for local conditions. A second caveat is that these reports are based upon the companies' own information, not an independent analytical source and no long-term evaluative information is available for any of the programs. The programs included here do not represent the full extent of employer innovations, but only a cluster that is available for immediate examination.

Regardless of the programs' variety, certain commonalities do emerge, and serve almost as rules.

1.   The top corporate leadership publicly "blesses" the program, either initially or at some propitious moment in the program's development. In some cases, chief executive involvement is direct and ongoing; in other cases, it is a symbolic gesture but nonetheless significant.

2.   Someone must be given authority and responsibility for the task. If the new program is just a subtask for someone with an already full schedule or if the person responsible does not at least have *direct* access to top authority, the project is headed for internal conflict.

3.   The greater the corporate commitment, the greater the rewards. Time, not money, is usually the scarcest resource.

4.   Although cooperation among employers is highly desirable, most companies have found that "going it alone" at the start saves time and produces a faster return on investment.

5.   The program should be designed for small but early success—new programs frequently die trying to do too much too soon. Success breeds more success if kept to a manageable level.

6.   Despite early successes, the real economic and health rewards are generally measurable only in the long term. This need not be decades, but it is a mistake to promise or expect major changes to occur with great speed.

7.   In nearly every instance, the corporation will need to develop and store new data in an easily retrievable form.

8.   Whether by promotion, hiring, or use of consultants, new programs must be supplied with more people and new types of skills.

9.   Government, more often than not, is an ally. New laws, regulations, and programs, however onerous, are also instruments of change which employers can turn to their advantage.

10.   The myth that medical care providers are the only ones capable of understanding the medical care system must be overcome. Business and

the providers can, and nearly always do, form a cooperative relationship. But for that relationship to have substance and durability, it must be based on the understanding that industry's role has changed from passive payer to active, informed participant.

The models that follow are not prescriptions that other companies should take on faith. They are guides to some of the pitfalls and rewards of a major commitment. Above all, they demonstrate how essential commitment is. Unless a large number of employers, acting alone or in groups, make a similar level of commitment, the role of industry as a major agent in our health and medical care delivery system will have a minimal impact.

Goodyear Tire & Rubber

Goodyear is a useful example because it shows how much can be done without bricks and mortar. Most employers are not ready to start their own HMOs or build satellite clinics. Goodyear built on leadership and commitment. These are two qualities any company can understand and strive for immediately.

The Council On Wage and Price Stability summarized its on-site investigation of Goodyear's approach:

> [It] is holistic in a double sense. First, the company is involved in every aspect of controlling costs—the costs of benefits administration, of unwarranted individual claims, of systemwide patterns of inappropriate utilization, and of building health care facilities. Second, Goodyear focuses on the system, not particular practitioners, hospitals, or medical procedures. The company's emphasis is on altering general patterns of health care delivery rather than reducing individual claims that may not be fully warranted.[36]

At Goodyear, the chairman of the board is personally involved. While at first this was more symbolic than active, today Charles J. Pilliod, Jr., serves as chairman of The Business Roundtable's Task Force on Health and is an appointed member of HEW Secretary Califano's National Health Insurance Advisory Committee. The director of Goodyear's Washington office, Rudy Vignone, serves as chairman of the WBGH, a task requiring large amounts of time and resources.

The company is self-insured for health services. This produces immediate financial benefits since it means Goodyear does not pay premium taxes or profits to a carrier or a carrier's marketing costs, and company funds are not held in a carrier's reserves earning interest that could, and now does, do to Goodyear. More important even that these financial benefits is the stimulus for direct involvement that results from self-insurance. Another benefit of self-insurance is the ready availability of all claims data. Without hard facts, employers are at a great disadvantage in negotiating with physicians and hospitals.

The function of health care management was recognized as distinct from employee benefits, personnel, group insurance, and industrial or labor relations, which are the boxes into which it is traditionally put. Goodyear hired Richard Martin specifically to fill the new role. Now president of the Summit and Portage County (Ohio) Health Systems Agency, Martin has earned a national reputation as an exemplar of business support for improving the health planning system for for integrating many aspects of cost containment activities.

A major problem for employers seeking to influence the local health system is the absence, especially in nonheadquarters locations, of a sufficient mass of employees to command the economic attention of providers. A significant next step in the chronology of industry involvement in health care will be the aggregation of employees from different companies in the same community. More and more, employers are discovering that such cooperation does not contradict normal market competition and is essential both for the accumulation of adequate data and for the economic clout to become a force for policy change. In the Akron, Ohio area, Goodyear has taken the lead and organized technical and financial support from the rubber industry for the health systems agency, as well as sharing data that contributed to negotiations with local hospitals that resulted in reduced average length of stay.

Goodyear has also financially supported PSROs so that the hospital care for which Goodyear pays will be subjected to concurrent utilization review. Martin is quick to point out that Goodyear is not doing this review, the physicians are. Potential cost savings are considerable: $350,000 for each day's reduction in an average length of stay in Akron.

R. J. Reynolds

The appetite for expanding the corporate role as provider of health care can be gauged somewhat by the reaction to a single *New York Times* story about R. J. Reynolds's development of their own HMO: within two weeks, Reynolds had received some 1,000 requests for information, technical assistance, and employment.

Among the key characteristics of the Winston-Salem HMO are its outpatient, full-service facility, and closed-panel, prepaid plan. It has 37,000 square feet of space and a staff of sixty-eight to handle the current load of 10,000 members. Membership, which is limited to Reynolds employees and dependents, is projected to be 30,000 by 1979 (a safe prediction since there is already a long waiting list). There are no claims forms since Reynolds pays all bills. Equitable provides insurance for away-from-home care and the company guarantees protection against catastrophic costs. Inpatient care is covered and provided by local hospitals.

In the purchase and development of the land, facility, and equipment, $2.4 million was expended. The "break-even" time is hard to measure, but they now estimate 18–24 months rather than the original 3–4 years. They are already at a utilization rate of 436 days of hospitalization per 1,000 population, which compares favorably with the previous Reynolds employee average of 900 per 1,000 and even the current 681 per 1,000 for Reynolds employees in Blue Cross–Blue Shield after an extensive cost containment program.

As a model for other corporations, Reynolds's experience has a number of distinct advantages and disadvantages. By any standard, its early record is one of success. Enrollment demand exceeds current capacity and employee satisfaction is very high. Another advantage is that the costs, both of physical structure and program development, can be clearly measured. The locality was sufficiently devoid of competing medical personnel and facilities that it will be possible to assess the health status and cost impact of the HMO. And, since demand has exceeded capacity from the start, it will be possible to measure the costs, pace, and effectiveness of growth/no-growth decisions. R. J. Reynolds has provided proof that a company—without government assistance—can develop a high quality medical delivery system that is accepted by employees and the local medical profession.

The primary disadvantage, from the point of view of emulators, is that the HMO filled a serious gap in the delivery system in the Winston-Salem area (nearly 50 percent of Reynolds's employees had no family physician). Therefore, it did not face the start-up problems that most other employers will find if they attempt a similar effort.

That is not to say others should be reluctant to attempt the creation of their own HMO. Many areas have gaps in their delivery systems, and the basic characteristics of the prepaid HMO approach are widely transferable.

> R. J. Reynolds believes that companies may as well form HMOs so they can at least control costs and assure a high quality of health care delivery for their employees. The company feels that the emphasis placed by HMOs on preventive medicine is of great benefit in human terms, and that HMOs work to simultaneously enhance the morale and well-being of employees, promote their efficiency, decrease absenteeism and downtime, and reduce annual expenditures for sickness and disability pay. . . .
>
> R. J. Reynolds believes that the most advantageous aspect of the HMO concept is that HMOs reverse the existing priorities of government and insurance providers, hospitals, and physicians by focusing the reward system on keeping people out of hospitals, rather than placing people in them.[37]

According to Reynolds, their planning, analysis, and HMO development has exposed certain features that are critical for HMO development generally and thus enhance Winston-Salem's role as a model. Their experience supports the rule of thumb that an enrollment of 30,000 is about the minimum size needed to provide economies of scale while supporting a full-service facility and staff. Although ten companies began with this HMO plan, only Reynolds stayed with it to conclusion. Single-company development appears more manageable. After completion, sharing among many employers will often be essential.

The impetus for Reynolds's participation came from need, more than from theory. As noted, 50 percent of the Reynolds's Winston-Salem employees had no family physician. The emergency rooms were being used as an inappropriate and very expensive substitute, and no family physicians were available for new employees.

Opposition from the medical community was forestalled by retaining the services of the past president of the local medical society as the HMO's medical director. Staff recruitment has been eased by the absence of administrative paperwork, availability of corporate fringe benefits, paid vacations, scheduled hours, easy coverage by colleagues, no personal malpractice insurance, and a first-class facility. Image is essential for attracting top staff and for member enrollment and retention. This is not just limited to the physical facility. A target of fifteen minutes waiting time is maintained, much personal attention is paid each patient to overcome his anxiety of receiving "factory medicine," and provision is made for extensive communication with employees. Reynolds's chief executive officer has given his blessing to the program. Initial enrollment was restricted to assure the high quality and good management of care.

Reynolds's commitment to the HMO philosophy is fervent, a fact that is also one of the major ingredients of their success. In Mr. Tudor's words:

> R. J. Reynolds believes that HMOs, by demonstrating this type of heightened respect for patient self-interest, will become increasingly well known, and that the majority of thinking people will want to join them. . . .

> Since those in the private sector are going to be spending big money for health care one way or another, it becomes incumbent on corporations to investigate the HMO alternative seriously, if for no other reason than to be in control of the expenditures. HMOs give business a chance to ensure a happy and effective work force, reduce absenteeism and downtime, promote efficiency, and reduce annual expenditures for sick pay. . . .

> R. J. Reynolds regards health maintenance organizations as the trend of the future in national health care delivery. . . .

> R. J. Reynolds stands ready to aid with such plans in every way possible, in hopes of matching the cooperation the company received during the development of its own HMO.[38]

Employers Insurance of Wausau

Owing largely to insufficient communications, the public in general and employers in particular have tended to think of HMOs as a single type of delivery structure. That is not the case. Because many of the oldest and best known prepaid group practice plans are closed-panel, this design has dominated both government and public attention. However, it is the individual practice association (IPA)-type HMO that many feel has the greatest future. The reasons are easy to define: no physical structure is needed and the participating physicians retain their existing patients, and vice versa. The IPA is a network of existing physicians' offices and professionals who need not be dislocated by a move to a central (some would say "neutral") facility. The IPA retains all the basic economic incentive advantages inherent in the prepaid concept. Further, the federal HMO law requires employers to offer qualified IPAs, as well as closed-panel HMOs.

Employers Insurance of Wausau is in the unique position of having initiated a major IPA and purchases its services for the company's employees. Predictably, impetus came from the escalation of health care costs (especially apparent to an insurance carrier); the personal interest of Employers' president was also a factor. Not unlike the other companies that have become directly involved in delivering care, Employers was seeking a method of holding down costs without reducing service, access, or quality.

> We spent five years in our explorations. With the help of our policyholders, medical consultants, physicians, institutional providers, and an interested and cooperative local medical society, we set about to put together a plan that would retain the fee-for-service system, that would allow continuation of all variations of physician practice from solo to clinic, and most importantly, that would have the potential for producing the favorable results achieved by the closed-panel type of HMO, particularly in reducing hospital utilization. . . .
>
> Incentives were built into our pilot plan for all involved to hold down costs. These incentives were balanced with others that were designed to promote rapid and complete recovery through quality health care services.[39]

Like the Reynolds plan, Employers' IPA limited initial enrollment to allow orderly development and cost analysis. Also like Reynolds, Employers has placed emphasis on preventive services and keeping the patient out of the hospital. Health education plays a prominent role. With the emphasis on preventive procedures even though there are no bills to be paid, each patient receives extensive reports of all diagnoses and treatments and their costs.

Essential characteristics of the Wausau plan include total "patient management" by providing benefits for outpatient and self-care, extended care, nursing homes, and home health care. This full range of eligible levels of care beyond normal hospital benefits facilitates transferring the patient to the level that is most appropriate and therefore most cost-effective.

The reimbursement system has the physicians "at risk", thus changing their incentives to foster a new cost conciousness. A special fund comprised of 10 percent of all physicians' fees is retained against the possibility of a deficit in the plan's overall budget. The physicians receive these monies and any surplus that may exist at the year's end. Providers must sign a contract for each twelve-month period to guarantee availability of services. The policy holders receive 100 percent of any surplus in the plan's general fund.

Peer review, even of ambulatory care, and extensive reporting combine to identify and reduce abuse and over-utilization by either the physician or the patient. Hospital costs are contained, in part, by an admission certification program and by having the physicians "at risk" for all unauthorized hospital charges.

Plan participation includes 94 percent of eligible employees and 80–100 percent of primary care physicians (with variation by community). The high level of employee enrollment puts pressure on the physicians to participate because their patients are asking for the program. The average length of hospital stay has been reduced by 46 percent from 7.4 to 4.3 days. Hospital admissions have been reduced by 10 percent, and annual hospital days per 1,000 people is at a low 469. Absenteeism owing to medical reasons has been reduced, and the IPA plan costs Wausau 21 percent less than would the same benefits in an indemnity plan.

According to Jacob Spies, the program is good for the insurance industry as well as the patient:

> We see the plan as an opportunity for insurers to continue their role as risk bearers and as administrators of health insurance, as an opportunity to set up, manage, and control an HMO, rather than merely to support and finance it.

Gillette

Not every employer will find the aggressive management of Goodyear or the Reynolds's HMO or the Wausau IPA suitable for its location, circumstances, or business style. That does not mean that other companies are left to an increasingly unsatisfactory status quo. An older program just recently receiving the attention it deserves provides Gillette with a total health care delivery system, including dependents as well as employees. The system has a progressive array of cost containment features working in supportive combination with high-quality care and continuous study of occupational stresses and strains.

The program addresses several of the major issues facing employers as they consider expanding their in-house medical programs. The full range of services is available free of charge to employees. Staff coverage is provided twenty-four hours per day, every day for employees and their families. This arrangement raises the possibility that the occupational physician can serve as a general family physician. Treatment and care are coordinated by a nurse practitioner who makes home as well as hospital visits. All the plant physicians also have fee-for-service practices, are board and/or speciality certified, and are on a medical school faculty. Confidentiality is assured. According to Dr. Greer et al., "the occupational health physician has the same moral, ethical and legal obligations to his employee-patients as he has to patients in his own private practice. Personal medical records are kept in the medical department and are not subject to review by management."[40]

The Gillette medical program's annual cost of approximately $700,000 is offset by savings which they estimate to be $1.9 million. In addition to those savings, Dr. Greer points to the "nonquantifiable pluses" that make the program popular with management and the employees:

> Control of hospitalization costs since ambulatory studies done by competent physicians avoid excessive hospitalization costs, and the option of instituting second opinion by Gillette physicians on the appropriateness of surgical procedures planned by outside physicians is available in questionable cases.

> Gillette's physicians do their own peer review by carefully monitoring one another's records for appropriateness, and can review bills for outside medical services if charges appear excessive or unwarranted.

> Outside referral costs are controlled because specialists on the staff have developed ongoing relationships with their patients.

> The health maintenance approach adopted by the Gillette medical department emphasizes prevention, early detection, and control of diseases which should lead to fewer advanced cases and, consequently, less absenteeism, less staff turnover, and less need to initiate expensive treatment modes.[41]

Of the 55,000 patient visits to the Gillette in-house system in 1976, 43,450 were for nonoccupational illness and injury, thus clearly establishing the "market" for an expanded care system within the industry structure. Gillette's program is a model of the integration of a large in-house occupational health program with the insured nonoccupational medical benefits and the normal fee-for-service community medical care delivery system. Advantages of all elements are retained and the integration removes many of the disadvantages that exist when these systems function separately. In the Gillette system, the employees and dependents can see the same physician in their communities whom they see in the plant.

In sum, the Gillette program provides an example of the benefits of taking a broad, comprehensive approach to the total health needs of a specific population. The program does not distinguish between illness that is job-related and that which is not, between executives' health and factory workers' health, between the physicians' responsibilities in private practice and in corporate practice, or between the goals of preventive programs and those of acute medical care programs. Consequently, the employee, dependent, company, provider, and community all benefit.

New York Telephone

The New York Telephone model is different from the others because it is a developing philosophy of total care rather than a specific facility or delivery system or interaction with the providers. Health care management (HCM), as described by Dr. G. H. Collings, Jr., is "a mechanism through which a positive effect on the real health of employees may be achieved while containing health-related costs and optimizing the efficiency of the health care system."[42]

Exhibit 4
New York Telephone Company's Health Care Management Program

Level	Where Provided	Objectives	Activities
I	in-house & community medical care facilities	immediate diagnosis & therapy; management & coordination of care	specific injury or illness focus (diagnosis, therapy and/or referral). This is the entry level for most who subsequently chose to participate in HCM. Participation is voluntary.
II	in-house	plan, manage, and modify a lifetime health care strategy for each employee-patient	gain the trust of the employee/patient; development of health and medical history; provide health education; conduct individualized periodic health monitoring; apply the principles of preventive care to the employee's life-style; supervise the lifetime health care strategy (a dynamic process that is never concluded); computerize patient data which in turn facilitates ongoing evaluation of the HCM effectiveness and provides the information necessary for Level III.
III	in-house	improve the health status of the full working population (80,000 at NY Tel.); evaluate the population's health progress and its indicators (costs, productivity, disability, absenteeism)	based on the collective data from Level II, epidemiological and biostatistical research is applied to the specific health problems of the working population; Level II managers use the research results to adjust their individualized lifetime health care strategies.

Adapted from material in: G. H. Collings, Jr., "Health—A Corporate Dilemma; Health Care Management—A Corporate Solution," in *Background Papers on Industry's Changing Role in Health Care Delivery*, ed. R. H. Egdahl, Springer Series on Industry and Health Care, (New York: Springer-Verlag, 1977), pp. 16–28.

This approach grew from New York Telephone's recognition that the traditional schism between occupational and nonoccupational medicine was no longer valid, and indeed, many would say that it never was sufficiently justified.

> There has been a broadening of what is meant by injury at work, first to include, in addition to physical injury, diseases produced by the work environment (the so-called occupational diseases) and then to include diseases that are not *caused* by the job but are simply aggravated or adversely affected by the job in some way. The truth of the matter, of course, is that any disease in an employee is influenced by the job. In fact, the health of employees who have no demonstrable disease in the ordinary sense is also significantly influenced by the job—or any other activity that occupies as much as eight hours out of twenty-four.[43]

The Health Care Management (HCM) system was developed as a method of addressing this expanding concept of corporate health responsibilities in our era of increasingly limited resources. It is not a program that is or will be acceptable to all within either the industry or provider communities. It is, however, an innovative, comprehensive effort to face many of the complex issues that are more typically left to speech-makers than to practitioners.

While everyone is talking about the need to make the individual more responsible for his or her own health and about the impact of our life-styles on our health status, few companies are aggressively trying to get their employees to actually become more responsible and alter their behavior. HCM encourages each employee to work voluntarily with the company medical department on the development of a "lifetime health care strategy," and then on the implementation and maintenance of that strategy. The accompanying exhibit (Exhibit 4) summarizes the three levels of care in the HCM program.

The Level I manager must "personally provide enouch clinical care to maintain the patient's confidence but resist the temptation to provide all the services he or she is competent to perform."[44] The focus of the corporate health care manager must be on Level II which is the zone in which employee's "lifetime health care strategy" is developed, data generated for Level III, and Level III research applied to the needs of the individual employee-patient.

In all dealings with community physicians, the corporate health care manager maintains responsibility for the employee-patient and must relate all outside care to the in-house program and lifetime health care strategy. It quickly becomes obvious that one of the great challenges but also one of the great opportunities of HCM, is the communication that is essential between community and in-house physicians.

Conclusion

The models in this chapter have two additional points in common: all are in a continual state of further development and refinement, and none is designed to eliminate the community health care system. The extent to which the models are successful depends upon how much they complement and reform the existing system by bringing new economic influences to bear, by increasing access to needed care, and by reducing the waste that now characterizes our public and private delivery systems. Difficult and challenging though these goals are, they can be achieved without in any way reducing the high quality of medical care on which consumers rightly insist.

Policy Recommendations

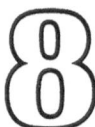

These recommendations are offered to catalyze further debate. All of them could not be achieved simultaneously and some may not be politically palatable. None, however, is mere fantasy and while I offer them on my personal responsibility, all have varying degrees of support from some of the industry leaders participating with the WBGH. The categories are arbitrary and serve merely to confer an order on the recommendations; I imply no priority among them.

Health Education

1. Congress should fund the Office of Health Education and Promotion.

2. Management, labor, and government should redesign benefit plans to provide reimbursement and incentives for health education activities.

3. In the same way, economic inventives should be designed for increased personal health care surveillance and responsibility. This might involve some version of the Breslow-Somers Lifetime Health Monitoring Program.

4. Industry should establish a coordination system to assemble, disseminate, and evaluate corporate health education programs.

5. The HSA planning review criteria should provide an incentive for hospitals to establish community outreach education programs.

6. A public-private research fund should be created to support the evaluation of health education methodologies.

Reimbursement

1. Industry and government should cosponsor the design and demonstration of a minimum benefit package that contains incentives for health maintenance, prevention, and promotion; basic physical and mental health care; and protection against financial catastrophy.

2. To the extent allowable by law, employers within the same community should coordinate their reimbursement policies and aggregate data collection.

3. Reimbursement should be designed to put the physician and other individual and institutional providers at risk.

4. Future benefit designs should include cost sharing by employees at a level that is not a barrier to needed care but that provides an incentive to responsible consumption of the health benefits. Cost sharing need not be exclusively in the form of deductibles or copayments; it may be in the form of innovative incentives to share the savings resulting from prudent utilization.

5. Health outcomes, rather than the provision of service alone, should have some bearing on the level of fee approved.

6. Methods and settings for care that are known to be cost-effective should be rewarded by the reimbursement system. For example: "If the insured utilizes ambulatory surgical facilities or extended care facilities in lieu of more costly inpatient hospital care, pay the reasonable and customary charge with no deductable or co-insurance."[45]

7. Physician assistants, nurse practitioners, and other properly certified nonphysician providers should be reimbursed for their services, either directly or through a physician. Physician supervision should be compensated only when it is medically necessary, but there should be reimbursement for the overhead expenses the physician incurs by the employment of nonphysician providers.

8.   Employer purchasing power should be used to stimulate a shift from retrospective to prospective reimbursement.

Planning

1.   The waiting period should be eliminated for consumers who wish to switch from another health advisory board to the local HSA.

2.   Experimental designation of insurance carriers as consumers rather than providers should be conducted. The carriers are now criticized for not being sufficiently consumer-oriented, but their designation as providers, offers little incentive or opportunity to respond to that criticism with constructive change.

3.   Government medical facilities should be included within HSA jurisdiction, granting that a portion of their patient load is national rather than local in origin.

4.   HMOs should be exempted from the certificate of need review until HMO development has reached a level where it can truly be said to be a health delivery system in competition with the regular fee-for-service system.

5.   The consumer majority on HSA boards should be increased to a level that will reasonably assure a majority at meetings. This percentage could vary from HSA to HSA depending on local preference.

6.   Training programs for corporate officers who serve on planning boards and committees should be designed and tested.

7.   The certificate of need requirement of P.L. 93–641 should be advanced from 1980 to 1979.

Quality Assurance

1.   Employers should work together to pressure the state and local medical societies and licensing authorities to enforce their own standards and disciplinary procedures more strictly.

2.   Peer review needs to be applied to all categories of patients and all settings of care.

Insurance

The commercial and Blue Cross–Blue Shield carriers are frequently criticized for not taking the lead in cost containment, health maintenance, and quality of care innovations. Their rejoinder is that their function is to respond to what their major consumers, the employers, desire. There is ample evidence that the carriers have occasionally offered well-designed benefits that were simply not accepted in the marketplace. Industry, it if wishes the private sector insurance carriers to continue to underwrite its health benefits, no longer has any choice but to provide the strongest possible market pressure on the carriers to provide benefits that do in fact meet the objectives of health maintenance and cost containment. The alternatives are self-insurance or government take-over. Few employers desire the latter and many cannot afford the former, so the time for concerted action to obtain responsive innovation from the carriers is at hand.

Programs such as second surgical opinions, preadmission testing, and concurrent utilization review must become the norm rather than isolated experiments. To be effective, these programs must be accompanied by extensive employee education efforts and be made a regular part of the utilization of the employee health benefit.

Conclusion

Countless other policy recommendations could be listed. Those above were offered because industry can actually implement or at least readily influence them. The list is a starting point only, but, if these items were implemented, we would have made major progress toward the development of a cost-effective delivery system with health as its objective and medical care as one of its methods. Industry can be the agent for change. It has the financial resources and financial incentives. It is just awakening to the realization of its potential. Industry should not be given the responsibility for directing change. Rather, it should take the responsibility for assisting in orderly progress.

This monograph has touched on many subjects. Throughout, there has been a concern for what we, as a nation, are going to do to ration our health dollars. This is an emotionally charged issue all the more difficult in an era of affluence and the public perception that medical care has become a "right" for all.

Rationing, however, is not new. It has occurred and does occur on all levels. When Congress funds an institute for one disease rather than another, that is rationing. Undoubtedly, people with the selected disease are better off and receive a greater return on their tax dollars than those who fall victim to a disease that has yet to capture the attention of Congress. The same can be said of administration policy. The major new emphasis on child health programs means there will not be a major new emphasis on some other worthy population category or research item.

Similar rationing is conducted by employers and unions when they negotiate to provide insurance for heart surgery but not for psychiatric care, or not for vision care or any other excluded treatment. Likewise, providers ration care for us as they select among alternative treatment modalities, or by their refusal (rare but far from nonexistant) to treat without prior evidence of ability to pay, or even by the allocation of scarce funds for one type of machine over another.

As individuals, we ration our own care by the type of insurance we purchase, by the degree to which we remain ignorant of our rights and options, and by the relative values we assign to shelter, job location, living environment, and nutrition as we make trade-offs in our daily lives.

It is time we stopped fearing the concept of rationing and began to face its reality. In the years ahead, limited resources, expanding expectations, new medical technology, and rising costs will inevitably force us to make even harder decisions.

The only alternative to the eventual allocation of all medical and health care resources by government is an immediate and continuous improvement in our utilization of the resources now available. We can do so much more with what we have that the ultimate—and unacceptable—level of rationing will not be necessary. Wiser utilization of our resources is what this monograph and industry's emerging role in health policy are all about.

NOTES

1. Lewis Thomas, M.D., "On the Science and Technology of Medicine," *Daedalus* 106 (Winter 1977), p. 44.

2. Robert Maxwell, *Health Care: The Growing Dilemma* (New York: McKinley, 1974), p. 7.

3. Willis B. Goldbeck, Washington Business Group on Health, Testimony Before the Senate Finance Committee, June 1977.

4. George Silver, M.D., *A Spy in the House of Medicine* (Germantown: MD: Aspen Systems, 1976), p. 279.

5. Sheldon W. Samuels, "The Problems of Industry-Sponsored Health Programs," in *Background Papers on Industry's Changing Role in Health Care Delivery*, ed. R. H. Egdahl, Springer Series on Industry and Health Care, no. 3 (New York: Springer-Verlag, 1977), pp. 152–158.

6. Ibid.

7. Greer et al., "Comprehensive Care through Physicians Serving in Both Corporate and Private Practice," in *Background Papers on Industry's Changing Role in Health Care Delivery*, ed. R. H. Egdahl, Springer Series on Industry and Health Care, no. 3 (New York: Springer-Verlag, 1977), pp. 48–57.

8. Richard H. Egdahl and Diana Chapman Walsh, "Industry-Sponsored Health Programs: Basis for a New Hybrid Prepaid Plan," *New England Journal of Medicine* 296:1350-1353 (1977).

9. John W. Hanley, Chief Executive Officer, Monsanto, quoted in Jean Briggs, "Toxic? To Whom?," *Forbes*, (September 1, 1977), p. 66.

10. Paul Oreffice, President, Dow, in *ibid*.

11. Karl T. Benedict, Sr., "Corporation Reaction to the Occupational Safety and Health Act of 1970," in *Background Papers on Industry's Changing Role in Health Care Delivery*, ed. R. H. Egdahl, Springer Series on Industry and Health Care, no. 3 (New York: Springer-Verlag, 1977), pp. 145–151.

12. Ibid.

13. Greer *et al.*, "Comprehensive Care."

14. G. H. Collings, Jr., "Health—A Corporate Dilemma; Health Care Management—A Corporate Solution," in *Background Papers on Industry's Changing Role in Health Care Delivery*, ed. R. H. Egdahl, Springer Series on Industry and Health Care, (New York: Springer-Verlag, 1977), pp. 16–28.

15. Karl T. Benedict, "Corporation Reaction."

16. Quoted in Roger Rapoport, *The Superdoctors* (Chicago: Playboy Press, 1975).

17. Quoted in *ibid.*

18. George Himler, "Foundations for Medical Care and Corporate Health Benefits," in *Background Papers on Industry's Changing Role in Health Care Delivery*, ed. R. H. Egdahl, Springer Series on Industry and Health Care, (New York: Springer-Verlag, 1977), pp. 103–111.

19. Henry C. Damm *et al.*, "Monitoring the Quality of Health Care Services," in *Background Papers on Industry's Changing Role in Health Care Delivery*, ed. R. H. Egdahl, Springer Series on Industry and Health Care, no. 3 (New York: Springer-Verlag, 1977), pp. 134–142.

20. Ibid.

21. Ibid.

22. John D. Blum, "Growing Legal Liability in Corporate Clinics," in *Background Papers on Industry's Changing Role in Health Care Delivery*, ed. R. H. Egdahl, Springer Series on Industry and Health Care, no. 3, (New York: Springer-Verlag, 1977), pp. 164–179.

23. Ibid.

24. Ibid.

25. H. A. Sinclaire, M.D., "Industry's Medical Involvement Today," in *Background Papers on Industry's Changing Role in Health Care Delivery*, ed. R. H. Egdahl, Springer Series on Industry and Health Care, No. 3, (New York: Springer-Verlag, 1977), pp. 29–39.

26. Ibid.

27. Quoted in Washington Business Group on Health, "A Private Sector Perspective on the Problems of Health Care Costs," a working paper prepared for the Honorable Joseph Califano, Secretary, Department of Health, Education and Welfare, Washington, DC, April 1977, pp. 28-29.

28. Ibid., p. 29.

29. Quoted in *ibid.*, pp. 31-32.

30. Thomas, "The Science and Technology," pp. 35-46

31. John Knowles, M.D., "The Responsibility of the Individual," *Daedalus* 106 (Winter 1977), p. 59.

32. Quoted in John Armer, speech to Employee Benefit Council of Northern California, January 11, 1977.

33. Ibid.

34. Ibid.

35. Ross Von Wiegard, *Business Insurance*, May 16, 1977.

36. Executive Office of the President, Council on Wage and Price Stability: *The Complex Puzzle of Rising Health Care Costs: Can the Private Sector Fit It Together?* (Washington, DC: USGPO No. 053-003-0025508, December 1976), p. 131.

37. Bynum E. Tudor, "A New Corporate Prepaid Group Health Plan," in *Background Papers on Industry's Changing Role in Health Care Delivery*, ed. R.

H. Egdahl, Springer Series on Industry and Health Care, No. 3, (New York: Springer-Verlag, 1977), pp. 70–78.

38. Ibid.

39. Jacob J. Spies, "A Corporation's Experience with Independent Practice Association HMOS," in *Background Papers on Industry's Changing Role in Health Care Delivery*, ed. R. H. Egdahl, Springer Series on Industry and Health Care, No. 3, (New York: Springer-Verlag, 1977), pp. 3–15.

40. Greer *et al.*, "Comprehensive Care."

41. Ibid.

42. Collings, "Health—A Corporate Dilemma."

43. Ibid.

44. Ibid.

45. Henry DiPrete, "Cost Containment through Benefit Plan Design," in *Background Papers on Industry's Changing Role in Health Care Delivery*, ed. R. H. Egdahl, Springer Series on Industry and Health Care, No. 3, (New York: Springer-Verlag, 1977), pp. 117–133.

Appendix

Conference Participants
"Industry-Sponsored Health Programs"
Boston University Center for Industry and Health Care
Boston: June 3 & 4, 1977

George J. Annas, Director, Center for Law & Health Services, Boston University, Boston, Massachusetts

Gregory J. Armer, John E. Armer Associates, Inc., Los Angeles, California

John E. Armer, John E. Armer Associates, Inc., Los Angeles, California

Cary E. Ashley, Director, Employee Benefits, Monsanto Company, St. Louis, Missouri

Karl T. Benedict, Sr., M.D., Norton Corporation, Worcester, Massachusetts

Richard I. Bergman, Executive Vice President, Systemedics, Inc., Princeton, New Jersey

William J. Bicknell, M.D., Medical Director, United Mine Workers of America, Health and Retirement Funds, Washington, DC

Peter A. Biggens, Manager, Corporate Benefits, Xerox Corporation, Stamford, Connecticut

John D. Blum, Research Associate in Health Law, Health Policy Institute, Boston University, Boston, Massachusetts

William F. Brownlee, Assistant Secretary, Group Insurance Operations, Connecticut General Life Insurance Company, Hartford, Connecticut

Rick J. Carlson, Mill Valley, California

Gilbeart Collings, M.D., Medical Director, New York Telephone, New York, New York

Richard Coyne, M.D., Director, Occupational Health, Smith Kline Corporation, Philadelphia, Pennsylvania

Edward Crane, Cato Institute, San Francisco, California

Henry Damm, Damm and Associates, Cleveland, Ohio

Stanley P. deLisser, Associate Director, E.H.E. Health Services, Inc., New York, New York

Harold Demone, Jr., Executive Vice President, United Community Planning Corporation, Boston, Massachusetts

Richard DiBona, Personnel Division, Employee Relations, Continental Bank & Trust, Chicago, Illinois

Henry DiPrete, Second Vice President, Group Division, John Hancock Insurance Company, Boston, Massachusetts

James Dockerty, Employee Relations Associate, Shell Oil Company, Houston, Texas

Richard H. Egdahl, M.D. (Moderator), Academic Vice President for Health Affairs, Director, Boston University Medical Center, Director, Health Policy Institute, Boston, Massachusetts

Stanley Finkelstein, M.D., Lecturer in Health Policy, Massachusetts Institute of Technology, Cambridge, Massachusetts

John Friedland, Research Analyst, Health Policy Institute, Boston, Massachusetts

Paul Gertman, M.D., Director, Health Services Research & Development, Boston University Medical Center, Boston, Massachusetts

Donald R. Giller, Director, Office of Informational Services, Boston University Medical Center, Boston, Massachusetts

Melvin A. Glasser, Director of Social Security Department, United Auto Workers, Detroit, Michigan

William Greer, M.D., Medical Director, Gillette Corporation, Boston, Massachusetts

Willis B. Goldbeck, Executive Director, Washington Business Group on Health, Washington, DC

Jeannette V. Haase, Assistant Academic Vice President for Health Affairs, Assistant Director, Health Policy Institute, Boston University, Boston, Massachusetts

Michael Herbert, Executive Director, Greater Bridgeport Medical Foundation, Fairfield, Connecticut

Thomas Herriman, Editor, *Labor Unity*, Amalgamated Clothing & Textile Workers Union, New York, New York

George Himler, M.D., President, American Association of Foundations for Medical Care, New York, New York

Daniel Hodan, Corporate Director, Benefits, TRW, Inc., Cleveland, Ohio

Frank J. Kefferstan II, M.D., Vice President & Medical Director, John Hancock Insurance Company, Boston, Massachusetts

William Koch, Koch Industries, Wellesley, Massachusetts

James E. Lapping, Director, Safety & Occupational Health, Building & Construction Trades Department, AFL-CIO, Washington, DC

Sol Levine, University Professor and Chairman, Department of Sociology, Boston University, Boston, Massachusetts

David Magnuson, Secretary, Corporate Affairs, Worcester Tool & Stamping Company, Rochdale, Massachusetts

Mark Mandel, Director, Regulatory Activities, Center for Health Planning, Boston University, Boston, Massachusetts

Richard Martin, Manager, Health Service Industry Relations, Goodyear Tire & Rubber Company, Akron, Ohio

William P. McHenry, Jr., Manager of Health, Coopers and Lybrand, Washington, DC

Joseph M. Miller, M.D., Medical Care Affiliates, Inc., Boston, Massachusetts

Judith A. Miller, General Director, Health Staff Seminar, George Washington University, Washington, DC

Barry Minkin, Manager, Group Insurance, SCM Corporation, New York, New York

Alan Monheit, Research Associate in Economics, Health Policy Institute, Boston University, Boston, Massachusetts

James I. Murray, Director, Insured Employee Benefits, Federated Department Stores, Inc., Cincinnati, Ohio

Thomas E. Parfitt, Vice President, Harris Trust & Savings Bank, Chicago, Illinois

R. Weston Pierce, Senior Vice President, Marketing, Blue Cross Association, Chicago, Illinois

Charles J. Pilliod, Jr. (Dinner Speaker, June 3rd, 1977), Chairman of the Board, Goodyear Tire & Rubber Company, Akron, Ohio

Harold Richmond, M.D., Corporate Medical Director, Columbus Occupational Health Association, Columbus, Indiana

J. R. Robinson, Manager, Employee Relations Department, Dupont, Wilmington, Delaware

Sheldon Samuels, Director of Occupational Health & Environmental Affairs, AFL-CIO, Washington, DC

Mark Schofield, Research Assistant, Health Policy Institute, Boston University, Boston, Massachusetts

Stuart H. Shapiro, M.D., Professional Staff Member, Health Subcommittee, Committee on Human Resources, Washington, DC

H. A. Sinclaire, M.D., Medical Director, Mobil Oil Corporation, New York, New York

Art Speigal, President, American Practice Management, New York, New York

Jacob Spies, Assistant Vice President, Health Care Systems, Employers Insurance of Wausau, Wausau, Wisconsin

Richard Sulc, Director, Health Care Consulting, New England, Coopers and Lybrand, Boston, Massachusetts

Cynthia H. Taft, Research Associate in Health Planning, Health Policy Institute, Boston University, Boston, Massachusetts

John Larkin Thompson, President, Blue Shield of Massachusetts, Boston, Massachusetts

C. Stephen Tsorvas, Consultant, Employee Benefits, General Electric Company, Fairfield, Connecticut

Bynum Tudor, Director, Corporate Employee Benefits, R. J. Reynolds Industries, Inc., Winston-Salem, North Carolina

Diana Chapman Walsh, Assistant Editor, Springer Series on Industry and Health Care, Health Policy Institute, Boston University, Boston, Massachusetts

Leon J. Warshaw, M.D., Vice President & Corporate Medical Director, Equitable Life Assurance Society of the United States, New York, New York

Glen Wegner, M.D., Medical Director, Boise Cascade Corporation, Boise, Idaho

Neil Weiner, Manager, Research Department, Health & Welfare Group, Central States Health, Welfare & Pension Fund, Chicago, Illinois

Victor M. Zink, Director of Employee Benefits & Services, Industrial Relations Staff, General Motors Corporation, Detroit, Michigan